New Wun Ching Developmental Publishing Co., Ltd.

New Age · New Choice · The Best Selected Educational Publications — NEW WCDP

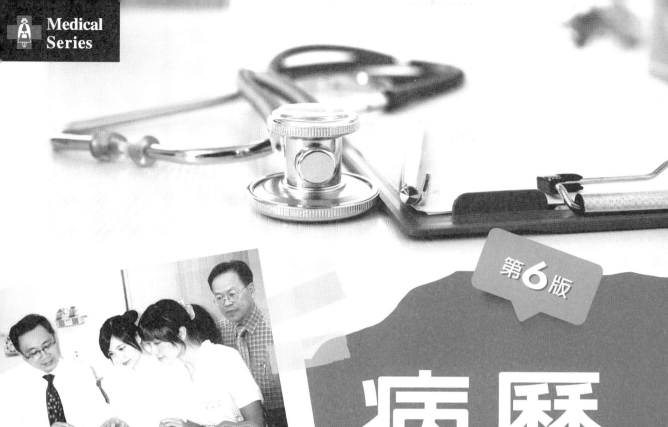

Medical Series

第**6**版

中央研究院院士
陳建仁

PROFESSIONALS
專業推薦
RECOMMENDATION

病歷+閱讀

Understanding Medical Records

➕ **審訂者**

徐會棋　胡月娟
李中一　鍾國彪
張銘峰　林清華

➕ **編著者**

劉明德　蔡玟蕙　郭彥志　黃盈禎　林玫君　鄭雅敏　徐玉珍
張　玠　陳寶如　陳勝美　薛承君　Jonathan Chen-Ken Seak
王守玉　卓淑美　李正喆　魏鈴穎　曹永昌　謝瓊慧　梁繼權
謝如蘭　張皓翔　潘昭貴　林鳳映　陳麗琴　陳麗貞　陳滄山
陳瑋芬　周志和　釋高上　王惠芳　李惠萍　李昭瑩

6th Edition

本書特色
Features of the Book

　　「病歷閱讀」是結合國內各大醫學中心的醫師與護理科系的教師，將其教學與實務經驗依病歷概論、內科、外科、婦產科、兒科、精神科、各科門診、老年醫學、護理記錄、電子病歷等主題，以常見的個案依序介紹病歷的書寫方式與閱讀技巧，讓學生能結合臨床應用的需求與培養英文能力，為目前國內最好的護理臨床教學書籍之一。

　　本書自付梓迄今，受到多校的支持與採用，特此感激。為使學生獲得更為完整的病歷閱讀技巧，第六版主要增訂方向包括：

1. 於各科病歷中列出「病歷小幫手」及「護理小幫手」專欄，讓學生能夠了解病歷中的書寫要點、病情發展、治療方式與相關護理措施。

2. 此版廣泛採納使用教師們回饋的建議，修正病歷英文文法之錯誤，使本書更臻完善。

3. 此版參酌臺灣醫療現況，新增老年醫學病歷，以因應高齡化浪潮。

　　本書的出版，對國內醫護人員的教學與指導可說能夠產生相當大的實用功效。特別感謝各界的回饋與建議，書中內容倘若有未盡之處，尚祈諸位護理先進及讀者能不吝指正，俾利此書能更臻於實用與豐富。

新文京編輯部　謹識

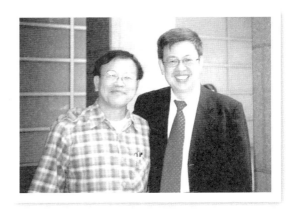

陳建仁院士（右）與劉明德攝於臺大

陳建仁
美國約翰霍普金斯大學流行病學博士
中央研究院院士暨特聘研究員
國立臺灣大學流行病學研究所兼任教授
曾任行政院衛生署署長

　　「工欲善其事，必先利其器」，正確而實用的教科書，是老師和學生必備的書籍。現有的醫護專用英文書籍，雖然琳瑯滿目，但是內容各有偏重的領域，適用於護理人員的英文學習，而且與臨床護理實務結合的書籍，相當少見。許多新出版的醫護英文書籍，或是倉促出版而有疏漏，或是未能兼顧實用性和易懂性。隨著醫藥護理科技的日新月異，如果培養專業護理人員英語能力的書籍不夠完備而更新，不但直接影響醫護教學的品質，也間接影響醫護人員的語文能力。

　　明德一向力爭上游，也積極關心國內醫護學生的學習成效。很高興看到由劉明德先生策劃，集合醫護及外文跨領域專業人才共同編寫的病歷閱讀之問世。這本嶄新而質優的教學用書，課程章節編排合宜，不僅讓讀者一目了然，更符合實際教學需要。本書內容豐富而條理清晰，可以看出編著者和出版公司的用心，可說是臺灣近年來出版的重要醫護書籍之一。它既符合臨床醫學與生命科學及通識課程的教學需求，並能增進醫護領域學生的臨床學習，值得醫學、護理、醫管（健康事業管理）等科系學生，以及從事臨床護理或行政工作人員一讀。我很樂意再次推薦本書，希望國內的醫護工作者能學習得更有成效，也給國人更安全更有效的醫療照護。

陳建仁　謹識

審訂者序
Preface

徐會棋
臺北市立聯合醫院陽明院區前院長
國立陽明大學（生理所及醫學系）專任教授
臺北榮總血液腫瘤科兼任主治醫師

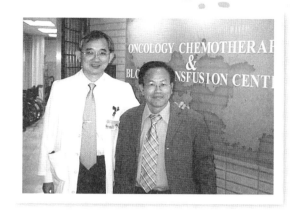

徐會棋教授（左）與劉明德攝於臺北榮總

　　時光飛逝，在我數十年從事研究的過程中，回首所受的臨床醫學教育，和我數十年來所教導的學生們，驀然發現，好的教科書絕對是一個課程，甚至是一個學門能夠受到重視並蓬勃發展最重要的因素之一。不久之前已問世的醫護英文用語及醫護英文－醫療照護會話篇深受讀者喜愛；此刻，再次由新文京開發出版股份有限公司出版，由劉明德先生與郭彥志醫師等人所編著策劃的病歷閱讀，看得出都是內容相當實在，且容易上手的好書。

　　劉明德先生曾在榮總跟隨我從事研究、並在陽明大學醫學系擔任了我的研究助理，一路所做的研究相當地踏實，而我發現這樣的性格，同時也反映在這本書的內容裡：內容整理豐富，且條理分明、井然有序。本書的出版，對國內醫護人員的教學與指導，可說能夠產生相當大的實用功效。因此，在翻閱過內容之後，我欣然地再次接受此書的審訂工作。我認為這樣內容實在的好書，確實是目前國內醫護教育界所需要的，相當值得推薦。

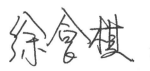 謹識

審訂者序
Preface

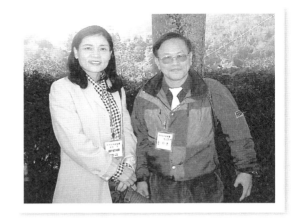

胡月娟教授（右）與劉明德攝於
臺大校友旅遊

胡月娟
英國歐斯特大學護理學博士
中臺科技大學護理系教授

　　劉明德先生任教於本校醫務管理系與護理系，也有與教學相關的書籍著作，包括：病歷閱讀、醫護英文－醫療照護會話篇、醫護英文用語、醫護術語、醫護專業術語、觀光英語、管理學競爭優勢（譯著）、基礎統計學（校閱）、普通微生物學、公共衛生概論、流行病學等。劉先生畢業於臺灣大學，雖然走入學術路線出道較晚，但他向來教學認真，頗受學生讚賞。最近他又回臺灣大學流行病學研究所參與升等研究，相信以他的毅力與勇氣堅持下去，終究會有所收穫。

　　劉先生在醫護英文用語出版後，並未懈怠，仍積極努力完成屬於護理人員在醫院臨床照護非常實用的病歷閱讀，可以看出他關心護理系學生將來在臨床應用的需求與培養英文能力的用心。有鑑於此，我欣然同意加入審閱行列，提供更多的護理資訊。

胡月娟　謹識

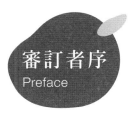

審訂者序
Preface

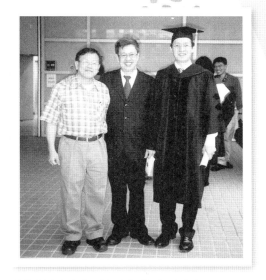

鍾國彪（右）、陳建仁院士（中）、
劉明德（左）攝於臺大

李中一
加拿大魁北克省 McGill University 流行病學與生物
統計學系哲學博士
國立成功大學公共衛生研究所教授

鍾國彪
美國約翰霍普金斯大學衛生政策與管理博士
國立臺灣大學健康政策與管理研究所副教授

張銘峰
台南市新樓醫院社區醫學部副部長暨家庭醫學科主任
國立成功大學醫學院醫學士

　　由明德與郭彥志醫師等人所編著策劃的病歷閱讀乃是繼醫護英文－醫療照護會話篇、醫護英文用語之後，為目前國內最好的醫院護理臨床教學書籍之一。明德和我們是大學同窗好友，畢業後雖然各奔前程，但我們還是會彼此交流學術方面的教學經驗。我們得知明德正規劃著這樣一項龐大又艱鉅的工作，編撰如此實用的護理人員臨床英文用書。我們當時便應允了明德邀請，為本書進行審訂。

　　在審訂的過程中，發現這本書的內容完完全全和明德的為人一樣，相當實際且清清楚楚。整理不但詳盡，在編排上也設計得別出心裁。以臨床醫護實務為例，明德等編著群將其敘述得相當活潑而不落俗套，著實有別於坊間其他相關書籍。這的確是國內教師和學生的一大福音，值得護理科系及醫護相關科系學生好好一讀。

李中一、鍾國彪、張銘峰　　謹識

審訂者序
Preface

林清華

現任凱旋醫院精神科主任
高雄醫學大學醫學研究所醫學博士
高雄醫學大學醫學系兼任部定教授
國立中山大學學士後醫學系合聘部定教授

　　病歷寫下了病人的醫療過程，閱讀病歷就是在閱讀病人從過去至今完整的疾病醫療史，藉此與其他領域醫療團隊溝通、互動，是為病歷閱讀能力乃醫護人員必備的技能之一。而由劉明德老師等人所編纂的這本病歷閱讀，亦可謂國內少數內容最完整、最豐富的英文病歷教科書，自其編排、主題選定等細節便可得知主編者的用心。

　　感謝劉明德老師邀請參與本書的審訂，但盡微薄之力，以使本書更臻完美、清晰明瞭，嘉惠更多學子，幫助學生及臨床人員學習更為順暢，得以學用合一，並將課堂所學完整發揮於臨床應用，祈於將來培養更多優秀醫護人員投入臨床醫療。

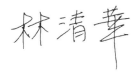

謹識

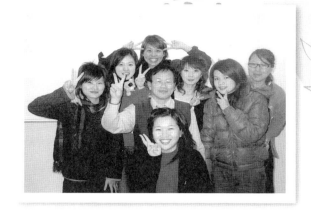

筆者劉明德任教弘光科技大學健康
事業管理系－醫學英文術語及病歷閱讀

筆者曾在弘光科技大學、中臺科技大學、聖母醫護管理專校任教醫管與醫護英文、醫學術語、微生物免疫學、病理學等課程，教學經驗豐富。在醫護英文用語出版後，為使護理科系學生在臨床實習對病歷閱讀醫學英文病歷、診斷與醫囑的能力，以勝任護理臨床實務工作，筆者與郭彥志醫師、薛承君醫師研擬出版醫護英文－醫療照護會話篇、病歷閱讀等書。期待這本與專業醫師及護理老師等人精撰的護理英文用書能造福莘莘學子，並於臨床應用，這是我們最大的欣慰與榮幸。

編撰過程中，筆者經統整各方寶貴意見後，隨即邀請教授群、醫護專業群及外語專業群共同編著，以做出有別於坊間相關書籍的實用工具書，使本書更添光采。感謝各位的熱忱參與，在此致上十二萬分的謝意！

此外，特別感謝推薦者：中央研究院陳建仁院士、審訂者，以及多位專業醫師的協助，其中另有病歷概論、外科、神經科、婦產科、兒科等入院病歷部分引用郭彥志醫師資料，使得本書更具專業應用價值！最後，更要感謝曾任中山醫學大學護理系林鳳映老師、台南市新樓醫院神經內科陳主任滄山醫師及時補齊神經科等病歷，得以順利出書，還有臺大學妹黃瑋婷協助，以及新文京開發出版股份有限公司相關人員的同心協助，並期盼任教老師及讀者不吝指正，謝謝！

劉明德 謹識

作者簡介
About the Authors

劉明德

國立臺灣大學流行病學與預防醫學研究所升等研究

國立臺灣大學微生物學研究所碩士（榜首）

國立臺灣大學公共衛生學系學士

國立臺灣大學健康政策與管理研究所演講「婚姻品質及生活品質」講師

現任國立聯合大學健康與生活、環保與生活講師

弘光科技大學健康事業管理系醫學英文及術語講師

中臺科技大學護理系醫護英文及通識教育中心環境教育講師

中臺科技大學醫務管理系醫管英文、醫學術語及護理系健康心理學講師

輔英科技大學應用外語系演講「跨領域醫護英文教學」講師

臺灣首府大學觀光英文、生物技術及健康科學講師

育達科技大學通識教育中心生物醫學、環保與生活、健康管理講師

聖母醫護管理專校護理科醫護英文與術語、病理學、（微）生物學實驗講師

仁德醫護管理專校公共衛生、（微）生物學、解剖生理、微生物科技與生活講師

考試院外語（英語）領隊人員及格

2015 年錯過升等助理教授

蔡玟蕙

國立陽明大學醫學院生理學研究所博士

國立臺灣大學學士、美國哈佛大學醫學院進修

現任臺北醫學大學醫學院呼吸治療學系兼任副教授

郭彥志

國立臺灣大學醫學系醫學士

現任長庚紀念醫院林口總院腎臟科總醫師

黃盈禎

國立成功大學護理學系碩士

現任育英醫護管理專科學校護理科講師

林玫君

英國 Napier 大學護理哲學博士

現任耕莘健康管理專科學校護理科助理教授

鄭雅敏

國立成功大學醫學院臨床醫學研究所博士候選人

國立成功大學醫學院醫學系醫學士

現任國立成功大學醫學院醫學系教授

現任國立成功大學醫學院附設醫院婦產部主治醫師

現任臺灣婦癌醫學會常務理事

徐玉珍

國立清華大學生命科學系生物醫學博士

國立成功大學護理學士、英國諾丁漢大學高等護理實務碩士

曾任仁德醫護管理專科學校護理科講師
曾任元培科技大學護理系助理教授

張　玠
美國猶他大學護理哲學博士
現任國立臺中科技大學護理系（科）助理教授

陳寶如
國防醫學院醫學科學研究所博士
現任亞東科技大學護理系助理教授

陳勝美
國立臺北護理學院護理研究所碩士
曾任國立臺中科技大學護理系（科）講師

薛承君
國立陽明大學醫學院急重症醫學研究所碩士
國立臺灣大學醫學系學士
現任土城醫院急診醫學科主任

Jonathan Chen-Ken Seak
M.B.B.S., International Medical University, Malaysia
University Malaya Medical Centre (UMMC)

王守玉
澳洲昆士蘭科技大學(Queensland University of Technology)護理哲學博士
曾任弘光科技大學護理系（所）副教授

卓淑美
英國艾瑟思大學(University of Essex)應用語言學哲學博士
現任弘光科技大學通識學院副教授

李正喆
國立臺灣大學臨床牙醫學研究所碩士
國立臺灣大學牙醫學系學士
中華民國口腔顎面外科專科醫師
現任臺大醫學院牙醫學系副教授
現任臺大醫院牙科部口腔顎面外科主治醫師

魏鈴穎
國立臺灣大學牙醫學系學士
國立臺灣大學臨床牙醫學研究所（口腔外科組）博士班候選人
中華民國口腔顎面外科專科醫師
曾任臺大醫院牙科部口腔顎面外科總醫師
現任臺大醫院竹東分院牙科兼任主治醫師

曹永昌
中國醫藥大學中醫研究所博士
現任臺灣中醫臨床醫學會榮譽理事長
曾任臺北市中醫師公會理事長
曾任臺北市立聯合醫院針灸科主任兼中興院區中醫科主任
現任鼎昌中醫診所所長

謝瓊慧
中國醫藥大學醫學士
曾任臺北市立忠孝醫院中醫科主任
曾任華夏石牌中醫院副院長
現任臺北市立聯合醫院中興院區中醫科主治醫師

梁繼權
美國約翰霍甫金斯大學公共衛生學碩士
臺灣大學醫學院醫學士
曾任臺大醫院家庭醫學部主治醫師
曾任臺大醫學院家庭醫學科教授

謝如蘭
臺灣大學醫學院醫學士
現任臺北醫學大學醫學系教授
現任新光醫院復健科主治醫師

張皓翔
臺灣師範大學生科博士
臺灣大學預防醫學碩士
臺灣大學醫學系學士
現任臺大醫院家庭醫學部主治醫師

潘昭貴
慈濟大學護理研究所碩士
現任慈濟科技大學護理系講師

林鳳映
國立臺灣大學醫學院護理系理學士
曾任臺灣大學護理系助教
曾任私立中山醫學院講師
曾任國立臺中護專講師
曾任私立中臺科技大學講師
現任臺中市大正診所護理師

陳麗琴
臺北醫學大學護理學研究所碩士
曾任長庚紀念醫院林口總院護理部副主任

陳麗貞
長庚大學醫務管理研究所碩士
現任長庚紀念醫院林口總院護理部副主任

陳滄山
中國醫藥學院醫學系醫學士
現任臺南市癲癇之友協會理事
現任臺南新樓醫院神經內科主治醫師

陳瑋芬
國立成功大學醫學系醫學士
曾任柳營奇美醫院神經內科主治醫師
現任臺南新樓醫院神經內科主治醫師

周志和
高雄醫學院醫學系醫學士
現任臺南奇美醫院神經內科主治醫師

釋高上
國立臺灣大學醫學工程所博士
國立臺灣大學醫學系醫學士
曾任國立臺灣大學附設醫院骨科總醫師、兼任
　主治醫師（教學診）
曾任新光醫院骨科主任暨骨科微創中心主任
現任新光吳火獅紀念醫院骨科主任

王惠芳
國立臺灣大學農業化學研究所微生物組碩士
高雄醫學大學學士後醫學系學士
現任羅東聖母醫院新陳代謝科主任
現任聖母醫護管理專科學校護理科兼任講師

李惠萍
慈濟大學護理學研究所碩士
曾任聖母醫護管理專科學校幼保科講師

李昭螢
美國華盛頓大學護理研究所哲學博士
現任輔英科技大學護理系副教授

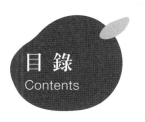

目 錄
Contents

01 | CHAPTER

病歷概論

作者｜劉明德、蔡玟蕙、郭彥志、黃盈禎

☑ 閱讀導引

1. 了解病歷的功能及重要性。
2. 了解病歷的書寫原則。
3. 清楚病歷的記載內容。
4. 熟知各式病歷記錄要點。

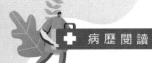
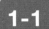 **1-1** 病歷的意義

一、病歷的定義及重要性

　　根據美國醫院協會的定義，**病歷是經由各種一般或特殊格式記錄病人被照護的資料**。病歷(medical record)乃是病人整體的醫療歷史，從病人的不適症狀、就診（門診或急診）到入院、住院期間醫療團隊成員依其專業對病人所行之處置或照護、病情進展，一直到病人出院為止。因此病歷是醫療照護中的重要記錄文件，必須詳實而完整地記載下來。此外，從病歷的內容應可正確辨識病人的身分背景、接受照護期間所得到的治療與檢查、保險給付的相關文件以及與法律相關的資訊，如同意書等文件。

二、病歷的範疇

　　病歷究竟應該包含何種資料呢？依醫療法的規定，廣義的病歷範疇包括：

1. 醫師執行業務時製作之病歷記錄表及體檢表。

2. **證明書類**：包括一般診斷書、甲種診斷書、兵役診斷書、死亡證明書、死產證明書等。

3. **同意書**：包括手術同意書、手術說明書、各種侵入性檢查同意書、侵入性檢查說明書、麻醉同意書、人體試驗同意書、自動出院同意書等。

4. **檢查記錄**：包括生化檢查報告、影像檢查報告、超音波檢查報告、病理檢查報告、心電圖等電生理檢查報告，或者檢查結果之影像等。

5. **病歷摘要**：包括入出院之病歷摘要、轉診或轉科部之病歷摘要。

6. **護理記錄**：包括護理人員照護之一般記錄、對病人實施之評估記錄、給藥記錄、生命徵象表格等。

7. **會診記錄**：包括會診各專科或社會工作人員、心理治療人員等，記錄被照會者之專業意見與處置。

8. **其他行政文件**：包括病危通知書、出院許可、外出請假單等。

三、病歷的功能

（一）病歷是病人照護的依據

病歷是記載醫護人員照顧病人的內容，因此所有觀察或檢查所得之結果均可在病歷上閱讀到。所以任何有關病人病況的變化也可從中取得，藉此評估當下病人適合接受何種治療。此外，與病人溝通的內容也應該記載在病歷上，俾使醫護人員能夠得知病人於治療上的期待，進一步使醫病關係更加密切。

對於其他專業人員而言，病歷是不可或缺的溝通橋梁，藉由詳細的病歷記錄可以節省許多聯繫時間，也可以避免誤解或遺漏病人先前的病況而做出失當的處置。在不同的專業之間，病歷是一種溝通平台，大家可以把意見彙整在病歷上，免除曠日廢時的討論，只需要定期召開會議釐清疑義即可。

（二）病歷提供教學和研究的功能

在教學醫院中，病人的病歷是提供教學的重要材料，從病人發病開始的種種病徵，接受過的檢查和治療，以及治療後的反應，都能讓學生充分認識某疾病的自然病程，也能熟悉處理某疾病的正確思維流程。此外，醫護人員將自己照顧過的病人資訊擷取重要的部分發表成為個案報告，可以提供同業遭遇類似案例時的參考，也可以彙整許多病人資料集結成為案例分析，或可成為業務執行上的一些準則；臨床試驗中，病人的病歷記載是統計人員所需的重要資料，倘若記載不實或不夠詳盡都會影響臨床試驗之效度。

（三）病歷記載的內容具有法律效力

病歷內容具有高度隱私，受到法律的保障，醫師非經病人同意不得使第三者知悉。與此同時，病歷也是記載醫療業務的文書，因此發生醫療或保險糾紛時，打官司的雙方皆可以依循法律程序取得病歷中的資料作為呈堂證供。詳盡的病歷記錄可以免除許多不必要的法律糾紛，在訴訟發生時也較能釐清因果關係，保障醫病雙方的權益。因此依醫療法第七十條之規定，醫療機構之病歷，應指定適當場所及人員保管，並**至少保存七年**。但未成年者之病歷，至少應保存至其**成年後七年**；人體試驗之病歷，應**永久保存**。

（四）病歷是保險給付的依據

由於病歷記載病人接受的醫療處置內容，加上病歷具有法律效力，因此病歷便成為保險給付的依據。根據病歷有記載的項目一一核對後才能確認給付的範圍為何。倘若病歷未如實記載，保險公司可以拒絕給付某一項醫療行為，屆時將造成醫院或病人無謂的損失。

（五）病歷在國家衛生決策上有影響力

公共衛生的研究常常需要藉助國家保險下病歷的資料，並且藉由研究大規模病人病歷的內容，協助公共衛生學者和醫療行政官員制訂更加符合現況及維護醫病雙方權益的衛生決策、行政規則。許多專科醫學會制訂的臨床決策指引也多需藉助病歷記錄中的資訊。這些病歷中隱含的人口學資料也會經由國家單位收集整理，發布成為國家級的衛生人口學資料，以與國際上其他國家相互比較，取得互相交流、截長補短的管道。

四、病歷記錄的書寫原則

何謂一本好的病歷呢？簡單來說就是要以最精簡的文字和圖形，將病人的就診與治療過程完整且正確的呈現出來。而每家醫院都有其對病歷的規範，但在記錄上的書寫原則仍然還是有一般的原則性。例如：

1. 病人治療或檢查後均應書寫記錄。

2. 病歷的書寫時間需掌握在適當的時間，不可延遲，並需註明完整的年、月、日。

3. 記錄內容必須正確、完整、簡明、清楚。記錄單張上的欄位都必須填寫，不要空白，病人的基本資料也都需具備。

4. 當病人出現任何突發狀況或出現新的問題時必須寫記錄，直到病情穩定或問題解決。

5. 病人所出現的症狀，都必須清楚記錄症狀情形、發生時間、期間及相關症狀等。最好以病人的口吻敘述，不要自行重新詮釋病人的意思。

6. 盡量少使用自創的縮寫，以減少爭議。因為有縮寫在不同領域所代表的意思又不同。

7. 已完成的記錄不可隨意修改。

8. 記錄後必須簽章。

1-2 病歷的內容

　　病歷最重要的部分是臨床記錄與行政記錄。臨床記錄主要陳述病人的概況，提供團隊和往後之醫療提供者有關此病人過往疾病的資訊；行政上的記錄則包含病人的個人資訊、法律相關的各式同意書及說明書等。

一、臨床記錄

　　病人的臨床記錄可以分為以下數類：

1. **病史**(history)：包含主訴(chief complaint)、現在病史(present illness)、過去病史(past history)、個人與家族史(personal and family history)、系統回顧(review of systems)。

2. **身體檢查**(physical examination)。

3. **醫囑**(physician's order)。

4. **每日臨床／觀察記錄**(daily observation note)：包含病程記錄(progress note)、護理記錄(nursing note)、生命徵象表單(vital sign sheet; TPR sheet)。

5. **檢查報告**(reports of laboratory examination and other specific diagnostic tests)：包括影像學報告、超音波報告、電生理檢查報告（如心電圖、腦波、神經肌肉檢查）、血液檢查、體液檢查等。

6. **手術記錄**(operation note)。

7. **麻醉記錄**(anesthesia record)。

8. **會診報告**(consultation report)。

9. **出院摘要**(discharge summary)。

10. **衛教指導**(patient education/instruction)。

二、行政記錄

1. **人口學資料**(demographic information)：即病人的一般資料，包括病人姓名、身分證字號、病歷號碼、性別、年齡、籍貫（出生地）、居住地、種族（在種族組成較複雜的國家特別需要）、使用語言、聯絡電話與住址、婚姻狀況、聯絡人等資訊。

2. **財務學資料**(financial information)：主要與病人擁有的保險相關，由於在台灣私人醫療保險尚不發達，主要以自費與健保兩種選擇為主；然而在美國私人保險制度是其健康保險的主流，此部分就會詳載病人的保險公司、保單類型以及可以支付的醫療項目等。

3. **同意書和授權書**(consents and authorizations)：同意書指執行醫療處置前需先取得病人的知情同意，而授權書指病人同意其病歷對某一方釋出，通常是他的保險公司。除病人授權之對象之外，醫療院所與團隊不得隨意透露病人資訊予第三方知悉。

1-3 各式病歷簡介

一、門診病歷

由於多數病人都是經由門診求助醫療人員的幫助，因此門診病歷是最常見的病歷格式。門診病歷的內容包括：病歷首頁、初診記錄及複診記錄。

（一）病歷首頁

病歷首頁的資料不外乎病人基本資料、食物和用藥的過敏史、血型以及輸血記錄。其中**過敏史及輸血反應尤其重要**，最好能夠詳載何種藥物、何種反應、處理後有無持續之不良結果等。

（二）初診記錄

初診病歷的記錄詳細度應比照住院病歷。初診記錄內容包括：主訴(chief complaint)、現在病史(present illness)、過去病史(past history)、個人與社會史(personal and social history)、家族史(family history)、系統回顧(review of systems)、身體檢查(physical examination)、臆斷(impression)或暫時性診斷(tentative diagnosis)、治療和檢查計畫(plan)、衛教(patient education)及下次約診(follow-up)。

（三）複診記錄

複診的記錄方式特別著重於病情變化或新的檢查結果，因此無需重複書寫初診之所有資料，而應該選擇性地重點式列出病人的活動性問題。其內容包括：

1. **病情變化或病人主觀問題**(subject)。

2. **檢查結果或客觀問題**(object)。

3. **評估**(assessment)：包含病況與診斷的確實性、上次看診時用藥之療效和副作用評估等。

4. **計畫**(plan)：包括此次用藥、額外的檢查、以及對病人的說明或指導。

最後要留意的是，無論是初診還是複診，**病歷最後都需要有醫師簽章負責**，如果是由實習醫師為病人進行初診，病歷記錄後也需簽名，唯仍需**由主治醫師再次看診確認並簽名複核**才算有效。

二、住院病歷

雖然各家醫院的住院病歷排放順序有些不同，但原則上會包括以下內容：

1. **住院病歷封面**(front sheet)。

2. **醫囑單**(order sheet)：醫師開立的醫囑可分為長期醫囑與臨時醫囑，長期醫囑為常規性的治療處方，臨時醫囑則立即執行的治療或給藥，執行一次醫囑內容之後即失效，常用於臨時突發狀況。**由醫師開立醫囑並簽章，護理人員執行時需簽名複核**。醫囑單是醫師與護理人員溝通的重要管道，也是醫療責任之所依。醫囑的下達需包含：(1)開立醫囑之日期與時間；(2)醫囑內容；(3)醫囑的執行時

間，例如用藥的醫囑需寫明何時開始用藥；(4)每日用藥頻率、給藥途徑和給藥劑量，給藥時如需密切注意病人狀況亦應註明清楚；(5)實習醫師在醫院開立的醫囑皆需有上級醫師簽章複核始可執行。

如**有電話或口頭醫囑，該醫囑需由醫師在 24 小時內補簽於書面醫囑單上。**此外，當住院時間很長或者住院狀況變化多端時，需定期將醫囑進行更新。如此，除了節省頁面，也可以提醒醫師重新審視所有開立的醫療行為在當下是否仍然需要，避免不必要的醫療行為。

住院病人初入院時，醫師將會開立住院醫囑，其內容包含入院診斷、病情狀況、病人的飲食、病人活動要求、常規之處方及檢查、過敏史、生命徵象之觀察頻率、身體上各種管路和造口的照護等。

3. **生命徵象表單**(TPR sheet)：除記錄體溫(T)、脈搏(P)及呼吸速率(R)外，有時會加上血壓(BP)，每日輸入／輸出量(I/O)和重要的用藥，例如利尿劑、抗生素、止痛劑等。表單上半部通常是記錄生命徵象的表格，以藍筆標記體溫、黑筆標記呼吸速率、紅筆標記脈搏速率。其他空白處則填上飲食量、靜脈輸液量、尿量、排便次數與糞便特徵、引流管引出量、體重變化等，這些基本資訊幫助我們了解病人身體的水分平衡，對心臟衰竭、肝硬化、腎臟病和休克的病人尤為重要。

4. **入院記錄**(admission note)：住院記錄包含許多項目，這也是記錄病人病況與相關資料最重要的一段，其內容如下：

(1) **主訴**(chief complaint)：藉由主訴可了解病人**此次就醫最主要的症狀和目的**，主訴應包含**症狀**(symptoms)、**發病時間**(time of onset)、**發病的快慢**(mode of onset)、**症狀持續的時間**(duration)；此外，主訴盡量以病人的語言為記錄，不要加入醫學專業術語或診斷性詞彙（表 1-1）。

(2) **現在病史**(present illness)：現在病史是對主訴更詳細地敘述，必須以時間順序（由前往後）推展，並且著重發病前後一些事件的關聯。此外，應列入病人先前的診斷、做過的檢查、接受過的治療，以及療效的評估（表 1-1）。

(3) **過去病史**(past history)：含括病人從小到大較重要的疾病或醫療情境，以及治療狀況。如：慢性病病人或系統性疾病病人應詳述目前接受的治療方式，俾使現在的醫療團隊了解病人的醫療控制情形（表 1-1）。

(4) **個人、社交及職業史**(personal, social and occupational history)：主要是與病人相關的資訊，如：發展史、教育程度與教育過程中出現的重大變化、職業狀況、婚姻狀況、重大危險因子、病人的嗜好（吸菸、嚼檳榔、酒精濫用等，若有，則註明每日量及持續時間）（表 1-1）。

(5) **家族史**(family history)：家族史主要能夠幫助醫療團隊了解病人與親屬間是否有遺傳與接觸性疾病，如：過敏、癌症、感染症、精神疾病、代謝疾病、心血管疾病、內分泌疾病、癲癇、痛風等。家族史以**家庭圖譜**(pedigree)呈現，可得知至病人三代的親屬資訊，如：年齡、與病人同住之親屬是誰、親屬存活與否、是否有特殊的身體或精神疾病診斷等（表 1-1）。

(6) **系統回顧**(review of systems)：系統回顧是為了補足病史詢問過程中可能遺漏的重要資訊而設計的，一般由頭部、胸部、腹部、骨盆腔器官，乃至於四肢列出許多細項，一般可以預先列印出表格再以勾選方式完成回顧，以便增加病史的完整度（表 1-2）。

(7) **身體檢查**(physical examination, PE)：身體檢查是醫師運用眼睛、耳朵、手，以及簡單的器械（如聽診器、神經槌、量角器等）對病人進行一套完整的身體狀況評估。身體檢查進行的方式多以身體部位為單位來進行，一般會從生命徵象和意識狀態做評估，再進行到一般表徵，也就是外觀看起來是否有任何特別之處。在一般概況評估完畢之後，就可以依循頭頸部（包含頭、眼睛、耳朵、鼻子、口腔及頸部）、胸部（包含肺臟和心臟）、腹部（包含肝臟、脾臟、腸胃道等）、骨盆腔與泌尿生殖系統、鼠蹊部、四肢、全身淋巴結、運動系統（包含周邊神經肌肉）、中樞神經檢查、精神狀態等（表 1-3）。

(8) **實驗室檢查及影像學報告**(laboratory and image)：可列出對診斷有幫助之各種診斷結果。由於電子病歷的推廣，此欄多可以從院內檢驗系統直接引入。

(9) **臆斷／暫時性診斷**(impression / tentative diagnosis)：根據上述資料所下的暫時性診斷，或寫出數個要釐清的診斷。此項將決定病人的治療和檢查方式。

(10) **處置計畫**(plan)：針對上述暫時診斷擬定的檢查與治療計畫。

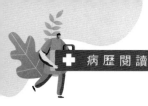
表 1-1　病史摘要

內　容	說明重點
主訴 (chief complaint)	了解求診的主要目的及其症狀
現在病史 (present illness)	了解主訴症狀之發生情況、持續時間、特質、舒緩因子、加重因子及伴隨之其他症狀
過去病史 (past history)	說明病人過去的疾病或醫療狀況，包含： 1. 慢性或重大系統性疾病：如高血壓、糖尿病、冠狀動脈疾病、腦血管意外、高血脂或血脂肪異常、高膽固醇、痛風等 2. 手術史：記錄病人先前因何種疾病動過何種手術 3. 住院史：記錄病人因為重大疾病住院的事件，可以和手術史合併記錄 4. 懷孕史：針對女性病人需詢問其懷孕狀況，記錄其懷孕次數(gestation, G)、生產次數(parturition, P)、自然流產次數(spontaneous abortion, SA)，以及人工流產次數(artificial abortion, AA)。此外，如有剖腹產(cesarean section, C/S)或其他妊娠期間之併發症如子癇前症(preeclampsia)，皆需詳細記載 5. 目前用藥：記載病人常規使用之藥物，包括：藥名、劑量、使用頻率及療效，避免與住院中之藥物衝突。此項可以和系統性疾病合併記載，便於查閱藥物對應之疾病
個人、社交及職業史 (personal, social and occupational history)	社交與個人史有時會和過去病史合併記載。其重點包括： 1. 婚姻狀況：已婚、未婚單身、未婚但交往中等 2. 菸：記錄吸菸之時間、每日幾包 3. 檳榔：記錄使用頻率及持續時間 4. 酒精：記錄使用頻率及持續時間。若使用頻率高、時間長，需評估酒癮形成之可能性 5. 職業史：記錄病人曾經擔任的工作、工作單位、工作地點及工作性質 6. 旅遊史：記錄病人近一年來是否曾到哪一國家旅遊或出差，這涉及一些傳染疾病的診斷 7. 寵物：記錄病人家中飼養何種寵物，這也和部分感染或傳染症密切相關
家族史 (family history)	記錄病人及其家屬之簡單健康評估，如是否有系統性疾病、已故長輩的逝世原因、癌症病史。最好能以病人為中心往上回溯一代，往下延伸一代，與病人平輩的，或是兄弟姊妹之健康狀況也十分重要

表 1-2　系統回顧摘要

內　容	評估重點
一般表徵 (general appearance)	是否出現體重減輕、疲勞感、發燒、寒顫、夜汗
皮膚(skin)	是否出現皮疹、皮膚搔癢、皮膚變色、皮膚結節
頭(head)	是否有鼻血、嗅覺異常、牙齦出血、喉嚨痛的情形
眼睛(eyes)	是否有視力模糊、複視、畏光、分泌物、紅眼的情形
耳(ears)	是否出現聽力損傷、耳鳴、分泌物
神經系統 (nervous system)	是否有頭暈、昏厥、癲癇發作、局部無力、感覺異常、記憶衰退、麻木的情形
肌肉骨骼系統 (musculoskeletal system)	是否有關節痛、關節腫大、肌肉無力、運動範圍受限的情形
心血管系統 (cardiovascular system)	是否出現胸痛、運動致喘、端坐呼吸、突發性夜間呼吸困難、間歇性跛行、四肢水腫、心悸
胃腸肝膽系統 (gastrointestinal and hepatobiliary system)	是否出現吞嚥困難、胸口燒灼感、噁心、嘔吐、吐血、腹痛、黑便、糞便顏色改變、黃疸、排便習慣改變、腹瀉
呼吸系統 (respiratory system)	是否有呼吸困難、咳嗽、痰液、咳血、發紺、胸悶的情形
泌尿生殖系統 (genitourinary system)	是否出現頻尿、尿急、排尿疼痛、泌尿道分泌物、尿液減少、間歇排尿、滴尿、排空不全、血尿、經痛、茶色尿
內分泌系統 (endocrine system)	是否有多尿、劇渴、細微顫抖、不耐熱、不耐冷的情形
血液系統 (hematologic system)	是否出現容易瘀血、淋巴結腫大、貧血
精神狀態(mental status)	是否有妄想、幻覺、情緒高亢、情緒低落的情形

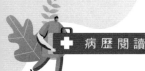

表 1-3　身體檢查摘要

內　容	檢查重點
一般表徵 (general appearance)	外表之健康狀況、外觀、身高、體重、衣著、衛生狀況、姿勢與面部表情、情緒反應、言語，此部分著重意識狀態之觀察與認知功能的簡易評估
生命徵象 (vital signs)	脈搏速率、呼吸速率、體溫、血壓、血氧飽和度(saturation of blood oxygen, SaO_2)
頭(head)	外觀是否完整、有無眼眶周圍瘀血、有無耳後血腫(postauricular hematoma, battle sign)
頸(neck)	頸部是否對稱、頸部是否僵硬，觀察有無頸靜脈怒張(jugular vein engorgement, JVE)，觸診有無淋巴結腫大(lymphadenopathy, LAD)
眼睛(eyes)	視力、視野、眼球位置和對齊性、結膜、鞏膜、眼外肌、瞳孔大小、瞳孔光反射
耳朵(ears)	耳殼、耳道、聽力、分泌物
鼻子(nose)	呼吸道、黏膜、鼻中隔、鼻竇壓痛或敲擊痛、分泌物、出血、嗅覺
口腔(oral cavity)	嘴唇、牙齒、牙齦出血、舌頭運動
喉嚨(throat)	扁桃腺腫大、扁桃腺化膿、懸壅垂偏移
胸(chest)	形狀、對稱膨脹、胸骨下凹陷、肋骨間凹陷、鎖骨上凹陷、使用輔助呼吸肌、呼吸音、異常／增加的呼吸音、震顫、叩診音
心臟(heart)	心搏、心音、心雜音、脈搏
乳房(breast)	腫塊、結節、分泌物、壓痛
胃腸道 (gastrointestinal tract)	腸音、壓痛、腹水
男性生殖器官 (male genital organs)	分泌物、水腫、病灶、直腸肛門指診
女性生殖器官 (female genital organs)	外陰、腺體、陰道、子宮頸、附屬器官
直腸及肛門 (rectus and anus)	肛裂、瘻管、痔瘡、腫塊、前列腺肥大、大便顏色
淋巴系統 (lymphatic system)	各處可觸摸之淋巴結，需記錄大小、質感、可移動度、是否疼痛、是否壓痛
神經系統 (nervous system)	顱神經、感覺系統、運動系統、協調、平衡、反射、巴賓斯基氏徵象、步態
周邊血管 (peripheral vessels)	周邊脈搏、周邊末梢溫度、肢體顏色、可觸摸之血管

5. **病程記錄**(progress note)：病人住院後，責任醫師每日需在病歷上撰寫病程記錄，而若病人住院超過一週，則需撰寫每週摘要，如因輪調單位離開病房或進入新病房時，則需撰寫交班及接班摘要。各種病程記錄敘述如下：

   (1) **病程記錄**(progress note)：病程記錄為每日撰寫，將病情變化扼要地記錄下來，其撰寫多半依據 SOAP 格式，根據每項病人的活動性問題列出：

     S: Subjective data，病人主觀感覺不舒服之處。

     O: Objective data，醫師進行的身體檢查、影像學檢查及實驗室檢驗等客觀發現。

     A: Assessment，問題評估。

     P: Plan，處置計畫。

   (2) **每週摘要**(weekly summary)：病人住院超過一週時，應於每週結束時撰寫摘要，簡單扼要地整理病人一週以來的病情變化、接受過的重要檢查結果，以及評估未來需要進行的處置和介入。

   (3) **交班及接班摘要**(off-service and on-service note)：當病人的責任醫師有所更換時應撰寫交班及接班摘要，以確保交班及接班的醫師都清楚知道病人的過去狀況及現況。

6. **會診記錄單**(consultation note)：醫療團隊在做最後診斷與決策之前，經常需要其他專科醫師的意見作為輔助，此時即可進行會診。會診單要填寫會診的專科科別、簡短的病史摘要、身體和實驗室檢查結果、影像學發現，以及希望照會該科醫師協助的問題。通常會診記錄之填寫包括：請求會診醫師的姓名和專科科別，會診理由（簡述即可），檢查發現，會診者的意見、臆斷(impression)或診斷(diagnosis)，會診者的治療建議，會診者簽章。

7. **侵入性檢查或處置記錄**(invasive procedure record)：侵入性檢查除了需要向病人充分告知風險、利弊與各種替代方案，與其討論並待其決定與同意（亦即需取得同意書）之外，尚需在病歷上記載此侵入性檢查的相關資訊。記錄內容包括：執行檢查或處置的時間、原因、方法、麻醉方式（如有麻醉行為，需要由麻醉醫師執行並簽章）、檢體發現及處置方法、有無併發症、執行檢查或處置的醫師（與監督的醫師）簽章。

侵入性檢查與處置包含：各種內視鏡檢查、血管攝影與血管內介入、可疑病灶之組織切片、體液抽取、侵入性高的血管內導管放置等。執行這些處置時需特別留意病人的生命徵象以及一些可能發生併發症的各種跡象同時記錄之。

8. **手術記錄**(operation note)：手術是一種侵入性更高的處置方式，因此更需要在病歷上留下記錄。手術記錄的填寫項目較上一項更多，條列如下：術前評估與診斷(preoperative evaluation)、麻醉方式、術式(operation method)與手術花費時間、術中發現(operative finding)與切除哪些部分、術中不尋常或意外的情形、手術器械與器材使用情形、術中估計失血量、輸血量、術中併發症之有無、繪圖以標示手術的範圍及重要發現、手術者與助手們簽章。

9. **麻醉記錄**(anesthesia record)：麻醉記錄通常與手術和侵入性處置記錄相伴，它必須包含病人在麻醉時廣泛的生命徵象記錄（包含體溫、血壓、心跳、呼吸速率、血氧濃度、吐氣末期二氧化碳濃度），麻醉方式的細節（包含使用何種麻醉藥物、劑量與途徑、給藥反應、術中是否補充其他藥物等），以及術後病人恢復情形（包含停止麻醉藥物的時間、病人自主呼吸的時間、病人接受拔管的時間、病人恢復意識和記憶的時間等）。每一張麻醉記錄單都需要負責該手術之麻醉護理人員與麻醉專科醫師簽字。

10. **給藥記錄**(medication record)：為整合住院病人每日接受藥物的情況，護理人員依據醫囑給予病人藥物時必須在給藥記錄單上填寫藥名、給予劑量、途徑、給藥反應、給藥頻率、給藥速率等資訊。倘若依據醫囑停止某項藥物之給予，也需要註明該藥物已停止給予。另外，每天負責給藥的護理人員必須在執行過每一次給藥後都簽章以示負責。

11. **護理記錄**(nursing note)：護理人員是醫療團隊中第一線的病人照護者，每天皆會觀察病人的狀況，同時對病人進行必要的評估，這些資訊都會記錄在護理記錄中，提供醫師對病人更深入的了解。重要的評估項目有：
    (1) **護理病歷**：於病人入院時完成，內容與前項醫師撰寫之病歷內容類似，皆包含病人基本資料、入院診斷、家族史、過敏與輸血史、個人健康史等。
    (2) **住院身體評估記錄表**：類似前述之身體檢查，但需每日填寫，作為每日監測健康問題訂立護理計畫與措施的基準。

(3) **壓傷及跌倒危險性評估表**：對於需要長時間臥床者，有糖尿病或其他壓傷高危險因子者、年老者、手術或侵入性檢查後病人都需要評估壓傷和跌倒之危險性，以事先預防併發症的發生。

(4) **護理計畫表**：護理人員依據每日身體評估和病人病情變化擬定主要照護的重點與執行的計畫，當病人病情與需求有所改變，新的護理計畫也會因應而生。

(5) **護理過程記錄表**：這是針對上述護理計畫表所制訂之計畫，撰寫當天值班人員執行護理措施時的狀況及病人反應，以確實呈現病人實際的病況和醫囑實行的成效。這些觀察和記錄可以做為參考，進一步影響上述護理計畫的制訂以及提供醫師更新醫囑時的方向。

(6) **出院規劃記錄表及出院摘要**：這些表單主要評估出院前應給予病人之衛教、病人自我照顧的能力、病人出院後家庭與社會的支持狀況、各種留置管路的清潔和置換方法指導、主要照顧者的衛教指導、出院時間等。

12. **出院摘要**(discharge summary)：本項係指病人先前住院過程之摘要。出院摘要著重於病人病史的摘要、住院期間進行的診療過程、用藥與治療反應、出院診斷及出院計畫。出院摘要的詳細項目如下：

(1) **住院與出院時之主要與次要診斷**：依照本次住院時疾病診斷之重要性依序列出，需要填寫全名和診斷碼。主要診斷指的是這次住院的主要病況，次要診斷則是原已存在或住院後才發生，並且影響住院醫療情況者；若無相關的疾病則不必填寫。

(2) **住院主訴及病況**：簡單扼要描述病人之主訴以及入院前的疾病進展概要。

(3) **住院治療情形**：本項目填寫住院時病人接受的治療計畫與治療反應。

(4) **主要身體檢查發現**：填寫入院時異常的身體檢查結果，特別是與入出院診斷相關的結果。

(5) **併發症**：住院期間是否發生新的病況，例如院內感染、藥物過敏、不良輸血反應、壓傷、跌倒等。

(6) **實驗室檢驗**：必定要填寫與主要診斷相關的實驗室檢驗依據，此外，住院期間重要的正常和異常數據也要列上。

(7) **影像學檢驗**：列出病人住院期間接受的影像學檢查，與主要診斷相關者最為重要，其餘異常之處也需列出。

(8) **侵入性處置、手術、麻醉及檢體發現**：重點式地記錄各項侵入性醫療行為及手術的相關事項。

(9) **病理檢體發現**：重點式地記錄各項病理報告結果、顯微鏡檢查發現及病理醫師之診斷結果。

(10) **出院狀態**：註明病人出院時之身體狀況，如：痊癒出院、帶有傷口或引流管路出院、依附呼吸器出院、自動或違反醫囑出院、轉至另一所醫院、死亡。

(11) **出院建議與出院用藥**：本項包括出院後的追蹤與治療計畫、出院後護理計畫、出院時應給予的衛教項目、出院開立之處方內容等。

　　出院病歷需於病人離院起盡早完成，通常在一週之內都不會被列入未完成病歷。完成的出院病歷可以做為病人申請保險理賠使用，也可以讓負責門診追蹤的醫師快速地在電子病歷系統中查閱病人先前住院之狀況，當然這也是醫院申報健康保險給付的最終依據。

三、急診病歷

　　通常急診病人的性質為急症或重症，例如昏迷、休克、外傷、瀕臨呼吸衰竭、中風等情況較為常見。

　　由於急重症的比例較高，面對急診病人無法像門診一般從容，病史的詢問也必須挑選最重要、最急切的部分進行確認；因此急診病歷的格式和門診、住院病歷迥異，其評估方式多從病人之生命徵象及嚴重程度下手，也可能先對病人進行治療，待穩定後才有機會詢問病史的狀況。

　　急診病歷的記錄要點如下：

1. **病人身分**：可由病人本身、家屬或協助就醫之民眾或警察獲知其身分，倘若不知道身分，基於救人之天職，可在緊急情況下直接進行必要之處置。

2. **時間點的記錄**：記錄時間點的原因眾多，特別與法律層面有關，由於急診室兵荒馬亂，等待治療的病人眾多，因此醫療團隊必須知道每位病人在何時進行過何種處置，另外也是為了保護自己免於疏忽。主要記錄抵達急診時間、發病時間、消防隊之緊急醫療人員到達現場的時間、來診方式（消防隊之 EMT 救護車、病人自行前來或病人家屬陪同）、檢查或治療起始時間（記錄醫療人員開始接觸病人並進行處置之時間）、離開急診之時間。

3. **檢傷分級之狀態**：記錄病人入院狀態是為了當作治療及病程發展的參考基準，要註明的重要資訊有：

 (1) **意識狀態**：清醒、昏迷或者介於其中，要詳細評估並簡單寫出病人對刺激的反應。

 (2) **生命徵象**：包含體溫、脈搏、血壓、呼吸速率、血氧飽和度。

 (3) **主訴**：病人來診原因。

 (4) **檢傷分級**：依據嚴重程度將病人分為五級，其中以第一級最為嚴重，需要接受立即處置。

4. **身體檢查記錄**：急診病歷多半印有制式之人體圖提供醫師標註異常之處。如有外傷或容易看見的病灶，亦可用相機記錄。最後註明進行身體檢查之時間。

5. **實驗室檢查和影像學檢查結果**：標註進行時間與結果。

6. **處置**：各項處置皆需註明執行時間與執行者簽章，以示負責。此外，處理傷口時需註明傷口處理前後的狀況，並畫示意圖描繪記錄。

7. **會診記錄**：急診的會診記錄需要立刻完成，並且書寫精確時間。

8. **病人動向**：於急診觀察或處理後病人的動向可能有住院、轉至 ICU、穩定離院、不穩定但自動離院等，病歷需記載病人確實的動向和離開急診的時間，若病人不配合醫師留院觀察的指示而自動離院，要在病歷上書寫離院原因並讓病人或家屬簽名以示負責。

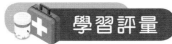

學習評量

( )1. 依醫療法第七十條之規定,醫療機構之病歷至少要保存多久?(A)五年 (B)七年 (C)十年 (D)十二年

( )2. 關於病歷的功能,下列何者敘述有誤?(A)病歷是病人照護及保險給付的依據 (B)病歷提供教學和研究的功能 (C)病歷在國家衛生決策上有影響力 (D)病歷記載的內容不具法律效力

( )3. 關於主訴(chief complaint),下列何者敘述正確?(A)可了解病人求診的主因及其症狀 (B)記錄時,加入醫學術語以快速了解病人病況 (C)以專業人員的觀察資料作為記錄 (D)主訴不需記載發病時間(time of onset)

( )4. 醫囑下達應包含:(1)醫囑開立時間 (2)醫囑內容 (3)醫囑執行時間 (4)每日用藥頻率、給藥途徑和給藥劑量 (5)實習醫師開立的醫囑不用上級醫師簽章複核: (A)(2)(3)(4) (B)(1)(2)(3)(4) (C)(1)(2)(5) (D)(1)(2)(3)(5)

( )5. 關於病程記錄(progress note)之撰寫格式,下列何者敘述有誤?(A)S, subjective data (B)O, objective data (C)A, action (D)P, plan

( )6. 有關醫囑的敘述下列何者為非?(A)護理人員執行醫囑時需再次簽名複核 (B)臨時醫囑的內容在執行過後即立刻失效 (C)為節省臨床醫師與護理人員的時間與成本,一份醫囑開立後盡量減少更新 (D)實習醫師所開立的醫囑需有上級醫師的複核簽章才可執行

( )7. 口頭醫屬必須於多久之內補上書面醫囑?(A)6 小時內 (B)12 小時內 (C)24 小時內 (D)48 小時內

( )8. 有關入院記錄的描述內容何者為非?(A)主述的描寫應以專業人員的角度與專業術語描寫才能正確表達病人的意思 (B)現在病史的記錄時間應由前往後推轉 (C)家族使可以家庭圖譜方式呈現 (D)系統回顧可補足病史詢問中遺漏的資訊

學習評量解答
請掃描 QR Code

02 | CHAPTER

內科病歷

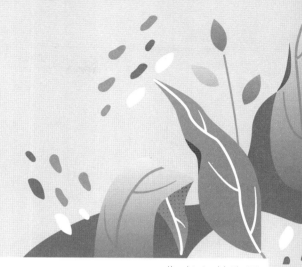

作者｜林玟君

Admission Note
Progress Note
Order Sheet
Consultation Sheet
Reply sheet
Discharge Summary

☑ 閱讀導引

1. 了解病人主訴與現在病史的關係。
2. 分析現在病史與過去病史之關聯性。
3. 分析現在病史、檢驗值與治療措施的合適性。

☑ PREVIEW

閱讀本章前，請讀者先自行預習糖尿病相關知識喔！

1. 糖尿病的發生原因與分類有哪些？常見的症狀為何？
2. 飯前、飯後血糖正常值為何？
3. 糖尿病的常見用藥治療為何？
4. 糖尿病常見的合併症有哪些？

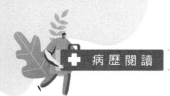

Admission Note

Internal Medicine, 60 years old, male, married, businessman.

Date of admission: 2023-1-1.

Chief Complaint:

Shortness of breath, mild fever, poor healing wound on the left plantar region for months.

Present Illness:

This 60 year-old male patient had history of type 2 **DM** for 5 years with regular medical control (Novomix 38 IU BID) and **OPD** follow up. The latest **HbA₁c** level was 12.2%. However, he suffered from mild fever with cough and sputum formation in the recent week. He also had the attack of urinary tract infection. Besides, he had one poor healing wound on his left plantar region, and his foot swelled in the winter. In recent 3 days, swelling, heat sensation, and redness were found on his left foot, and he felt fatigue with poor appetite, therefore, he visited our OPD this morning, where BS>500 mg/dL was noticed. He was then referred to our **ER**, where a series of **LAB** examinations disclosed **leukocytosis**, **hyperglycemia** (BS=673 mg/dL), acute on chronic renal failure, **hyponatremia**, mild **hyperkalemia**, and markedly elevated **CRP** level. Urine examination showed **pyuria** with bacteria (++). Thus, he was admitted to our ward for further management.

Past History:

1. **HCVD** and **Af** with medical control (Urosin 1# PO QN, Fedil 1# PO QD).

2. The history of major operation: Diabetic **retinopathy**, **OS** **s/p** OP, and **cataract** **OS** **s/p** OP.

3. No known food or drug allergy.

關鍵字彙 Keywords

字　彙	原　文	中　譯
DM	diabetes mellitus	糖尿病
OPD	outpatient department	門診
HbA$_{1c}$	glycated hemoglobin	糖化血色素
BS	blood sugar	血糖
ER	emergency room	急診
LAB	laboratory	實驗室
Leukocytosis	leuko- white，白的 cyto- cell，細胞 -osis （病的）狀態	白血球增多
Hyperglycemia	hyper- high，高、亢進 glyco- sugar，糖 -emia blood，與血液有關	高血糖
Hyponatremia	hypo- low，少、低	低血鈉症
Hyperkalemia		高血鉀症
CRP	C-reactive protein	C-反應蛋白
Pyuria	py- pus，膿 -uria urine，尿	膿尿
HCVD	hypertensive cardiovascular disease	高血壓性心臟血管疾病
Af	atrial fibrillation	心房纖維顫動
Retinopathy	retin-，視網膜 -pathy，病變	視網膜病變
OS	L. *oculus sinister*, left eye	左眼
s/p	post-surgical	術後
Cataract		白內障

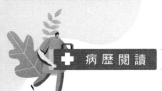

Personal History:

1. Habit of smoking: Denied.

2. Habit of alcohol drinking: Denied.

3. The history of occupation disease: Nil.

4. The history of traveling in recent 3 months: Denied.

5. The history of drug abuse: Denied.

Family History:

Family history is nothing in particular.

Review of Systems:

Throughout the whole course of present illness, the patient also suffered from symptoms mentioned as below: Chills(-), fever(+), night sweating(-), cough(+), sputum(+), hemoptysis(-), epistaxis(-), chest tightness(-), chest pain(-), **SOB**(+), exertional dyspnea(-), orthopnea(-), abdominal pain(-), anorexia(+), dysphagia(-), nausea(-), vomiting(-), constipation(-), diarrhea(-), hematemesis(-), hematochezia(-), melena(-), dysuria(-), oligouria(-), body weight loss(-).

1. Vital signs: **BT**: 37.6°C, **PR**: 82/min, **RR**: 24~26/min, **BP**: 142/86 mmHg.

2. Height: 171 cm, Weight: 76 kg.

3. Conscious: Alert.

4. Mentality: Intact to **JOMAC**.

5. Skin: No **petechiae** or **ecchymosis**, dry skin turgor.

6. **HEENT**: Grossly normal, no pale conjunctiva or icteric sclera, pupil with **LR**(+), **OU**.

7. Neck: Supple, no **JVE**, no goiter.

8. Chest: Symmetrical and free expansion, breathing sound(+), **bil.**, **rhonchi**.

9. Heart: Regular heart beat, no **murmur**, no heave or no thrill.

10. Abdomen: Soft and flat, normoactive bowel sound, no shifting dullness, no tenderness or rebounding pain.

11. Back: No spine deformity, no **CV angle** knocking pain.

12. Extremities: Freely movable, no deformity or **pitting edema**, one chronic ulcer over his left plantar region about 3×3 cm² and deep to muscle layer.

13. Neurological: **Hypoesthesia** of limbs.

關鍵字彙 Keywords

字　彙	原　文	中　譯
SOB	shortness of breath	呼吸短促
BT	body temperature	體溫
PR	pulse rate	脈搏
RR	respiratory rate	呼吸速率
BP	blood pressure	血壓
JOMAC	judgment, orientation, memory, attention, calculus	判斷力、定向感、記憶力、注意力、計算力
Petechiae		瘀點
Ecchymosis		瘀斑
HEENT	head, eye, ear, nose, throat	頭、眼、耳、鼻、喉
LR	light reflex	光反射
OU	L. *oculus unitas*, both eyes	雙眼
JVE	jugular vein engorgement	頸靜脈怒張〔表示右心房壓力升高和靜脈回流受阻（靜脈壓增高），常見於右心衰竭、心包炎、心包積液或上腔靜脈阻塞〕
bil.	bilateral	雙側
Rhonchi		乾囉音
Murmur		心雜音
CV angle		肋脊角
Pitting edema		凹陷性水腫
Hypoesthesia	hypo- low，少、低下 -esthesia，感覺	感覺遲緩

Laboratory:

1. Blood Gas Analysis

Date	pH	PCO_2	PO_2	BE	HCO_3^-
2023/1/1	7.333	40.6 mmHg	32.1 mmHg	−4.8 mmol/L	21.1 mmol/L

2. BCS

Date	Glucose PC	BUN	Creatinine	AST	ALK-P	Albumin	Sodium	Potassium	CRP
2023/1/1	589 mg/dL	36 mg/dL	2.1 mg/dL	10 U/L	70 U/L	3.5 g/dL	134 mEq/L	5.5 mEq/L	16 mg/dL

3. CBC

Date	WBC	RBC	Hb	Hct	MCV	PLT	Neutrophils	Monocytes	Basophils
2023/1/1	14,400 μL	$4.39×10^6$/μL	14 g/dL	41%	87 fL	292,000 μL	70.2%	7.5%	2.4%

4. Urine Routine

Date	Acetone	OB	Pro	Bil	S.G	pH	Nit	RBC	WBC	Bacteria
2023/1/1	1+	1+	+	−	1.019	5.0	−	20~30	>100/HPF	++

護理小幫手

Little Helper

糖化血色素(HbA₁c)

　　人體血液中的紅血球含有血色素，當血液中的葡萄糖進入紅血球，和血紅素結合後，就形成糖化血色素。一般紅血球平均壽命為 120 天，葡萄糖附在血色素上不易脫落，因此檢查血中糖化血色素的濃度，可以反映體內最近 2~3 個月的血糖控制情況。

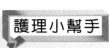

護理小幫手

Little Helper

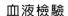

血液檢驗

- pH：7.35~7.45，偏低者表示與酸血症相關。
- PO_2：80~100 mmHg，偏低者表示與肺部機能及代謝狀況相關。
- BE：±2，偏低者表示與酸血症相關。
- HCO_3^-：22~26 mmol/L，偏低者表示與酸中毒相關。
- Glucose PC：應小於 140 mg/dL，偏高者表示與糖尿病、胰島素分泌不足相關。
- BUN：5~20 mg/dL，偏高者表示與脫水、大量出血、休克相關。
- Creatinine：0.7~1.3 mg/dL，偏高者表示與腎臟功能喪失相關。
- Sodium：135~150 mmol/L，偏低者表示與嘔吐、腹瀉、糖尿症昏迷、尿毒症相關。
- Potassium：3.5~5.3 mmol/L，偏高者表示與尿毒症有關。溶血也會造成鉀離子升高。
- CRP：<1 mg/dL，偏高者表示與細菌感染及急性癌症反應相關。

尿液檢驗

- Acetone：呈陰性，若有出現(+)，表示體內缺乏胰島素，而燃燒脂肪所產生的代謝物；糖尿病、饑餓、腹瀉、嘔吐相關。
- OB：正常應呈陰性，呈陽性可能與腎臟發炎、尿道結石有關；生理期婦女或服用維生素 C 也會造成誤差相關。
- Pro：若有出現(+)，表示與生理性蛋白（常見青少年）、腎病、發高燒相關。
- RBC：正常為 0~3，若有出現(+)，可能為腎臟發炎、尿道結石；生理期婦女會造成誤差相關。
- WBC：正常為 0~3，正常應無白血球或少量存在。若有出現(+)，往往暗示著泌尿道可能有感染。
- Bacteria：若有出現(+)，表示尿路感染或尿置放過久。

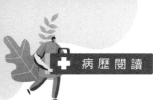

Radiology & Imaging Reports:

2023-1-1 Echocardiography:

LV-D: 52 (40~56) mm **LA**: 40 (25~40) mm **PA** systolic pressure: 28 mmHg

LV-S: 34 (20~38) mm **AO**: 34 (22~40) mm **Pericardial effusion**: 0 mm^3

IVS: 10 (7~12) mm **RV**: 26 (21~27) mm Quality: Good

LVPW: 8 (7~11) mm **RVW**: 6 (5~8) mm

LV function: Normal RV function: Normal

Structure: **MV: N** **TV**: N **AV**: N **PV**: N

Regurgitation grading: 1/3 1/3 1/3 1/3

- The left atrium is dilated.
- Mild mitral regurgitation is present.
- Mild tricuspid regurgitation is present.
- Mild pulmonary regurgitation is present.
- The left ventricle is normal in systolic function.
- The **ejection fraction** of left ventricle is estimated 70%.

2023-1-1 CXR:

1. Mild increased lung marking over bilateral lung fields.
2. Both lungs **parenchyma** showed normal appearance without evidence of focal mass lesion.
3. Normal distribution of the pulmonary vessels was noted.
4. The heart size was within normal limit.
5. The bony structures, including bilateral ribs, scapula, clavicles and vertebral bodies, showed normal appearance without evidence of fracture.

2023-1-1 Foot, L'T X-ray:

1. Deformity, **erosion** and degenerative change of the left plantar region is identified.
2. Mild **osteoporosis**.
3. No other remarkable abnormality is seen.

關鍵字彙 Keywords

字　彙	原　文	中　譯
Echocardiography	echo-，反響 cardio-　heart，心臟 -graphy，攝影	心臟超音波
LV-D	left ventricle - diastolic	左心室－舒張
LA	left atrium	左心房
PA	pulmonary artery	肺動脈
LV-S	left ventricle- systolic	左心室－收縮
AO	aortic opening	主動脈開口
Pericardial effusion	peri-，周圍	心包積水
IVS	interventricular septum	心室中隔
RV	right ventricle	右心室
LVPW	left ventricle posterior wall	左心室後壁
RVW	right ventricular wall	右心室壁
MV	mitral valve	二尖瓣
N	normal	正常
TV	tricuspid valve	三尖瓣
AV	aortic valve	主動脈瓣
PV	pulmonary valve	肺動脈瓣
Regurgitation	re-，再、回	回流、倒流
Ejection fraction (EF)		射血比率
CXR	chest X-ray	胸腔Ｘ光攝影
Parenchyma		實質
Erosion		糜爛
Osteoporosis	osteo-　bone，骨	骨質疏鬆

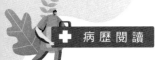

Impression:

1. Type 2 diabetes mellitus with poor control.
2. DM foot, left with secondary infection with **sepsis**.
3. HCVD.
4. **URI**.
5. Hyponatremia/Hyperkalemia.
6. Acute on chronic renal failure, suspected sepsis related.
7. **UTI**.

Diagnostic Plans:

1. Blood culture and wound **discharge** culture.
2. Check HbA$_{1c}$.
3. Arrange **PT**, arrange cardiac echography.

Therapeutic Plans:

1. Novomix dose adjustment, monitor blood glucose Q4H, **I/O** and vital signs QID.
2. Change dressing, antibiotics with Oxacillin and Unasyn.
3. **PS** and Chest consultation.

Educational Plans:

1. Explain to the families about the condition and prognosis.
2. Diet therapy and arrange **dietitian** consultation.
3. Arrange diabetes education consultation.
4. Adequate exercise programs.

Attending Physician:×××

Resident:△△△

關鍵字彙 Keywords

字　彙	原　文	中　譯
Sepsis		敗血症
URI	upper respiratory infection	上呼吸道感染
UTI	urinary tract infection	泌尿道感染
Discharge		分泌物、出院
PT	prothrombin time	凝血酶原時間
I/O	intake/output	輸入／輸出
PS	plastic surgery	整形外科
Dietitian		營養師

 Thinking About

1. 個案此次入院與糖尿病有相關的主要原因有哪些？
2. 請問主治醫師的治療性計畫的依據，可從何處判斷？
3. 請問為何醫師要個案會診整形外科？

護理小幫手

Little Helper

 射血比率(Ejection fraction)

　　指心室收縮時射出的血量比率，用以評斷心室收縮的功能，正常值為55~70%。射血比率與心肌的收縮能力有關，心肌收縮能力越強，則輸出量越多，射血比率也越大。

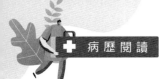

Progress Note

Internal Medicine, 60 years old, male, married, businessman.
Date of admission: 2023-1-1.

2023-1-2 10:30 am

#1 Type 2 DM

O:

1. 2023-1-1 9am Blood sugar: 568 mg/dL.
2. 2023-1-1 1pm Blood sugar: 466 mg/dL.
3. 2023-1-1 5pm Blood sugar: 426 mg/dL.

A: Type 2 DM.

P:

1. Check blood sugar QID/AC and PRN.
2. Control blood sugar with Insulatard.
3. Full diet, 1,500 kcal/day.

#2 DM foot, left

S: Painful sensation over left plantar region.

O: One chronic ulcer is over his left plantar region about 3×3 cm^2 and deep to the muscle layer. The appearance of the wound is red and swollen, with lots of yellowish discharge and feelings of pain.

A: DM foot, left with secondary infection with sepsis.

P:

1. Change dressing of the wound BID.
2. Consult PS for further treatment.

＃3 UTI

S: Mild fever, on and off.

O:

1. Vital signs: BT: 37.6°C, PR: 82/min, RR: 24~26/min, BP: 142/86 mmHg.
2. I/O: 850/1050 (-200).
3. 2023-1-1 **CBC** showed WBC: 14,400(↑), **SMA** showed BUN/Cr.: 36/2.1 mg/dL(↑), Na: 134 mmol/L(↓), K: 5.5 mmol/L.
4. 2023-1-1 U/A showed WBC >100/HPF; bacteria(++).

A: UTI.

P: Antibiotics therapy.

＃4 URI

S:

1. Yellowish sputum was noted.
2. Shortness of breath, on and off.

O:

1. Vital signs: BT: 37.6°C, PR: 82/min, RR: 24~26/min, BP: 142/86 mmHg.
2. Consciousness: Clear.
3. Heart sound: **RHB**.
4. Breathing sound: Rhonchi over bilateral lung field.

A: URI, suspected **pneumonia**.

P:

1. Antibiotics therapy.
2 Enhance **CPT**.
3. Oral medication usage.

Attending Physician: ×××

Resident: △△△

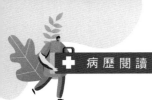
 關鍵字彙 Keywords

字 彙	原 文	中 譯
AC	L. *ante cibum*, before meals	飯前
PRN	L. *pro re nate*, whenever necessary	需要時
CBC	complete blood count	全血球計數
SMA	sequential multiple analysis (serum electrolytes)	連續多重性分析法（血漿電解質）、生化檢查
RHB	regular heart beat	規則心跳
Pneumonia	pneumo-　lung，肺	肺炎
CPT	chest physiotherapy physio-，物理 -therapy，治療	胸腔物理治療

Order Sheet

Internal Medicine, 60 years old, male, married, businessman.

Date of admission: 2023-1-1.

Standing Order

2023-1-1

Diagnosis:

1. Type 2 diabetes mellitus with poor control.

2. DM foot, left with secondary infection with sepsis.

3. HCVD.

4. URI.

5. Hyponatremia/Hyperkalemia.

6. Acute on chronic renal failure, suspected sepsis related.

7. UTI.

Activity: Bed rest.

Allergies: Unknown.

Take BP, PR, RR **QID**.

Record I/O **QD**.

Check blood sugar QID/AC & PRN.

Medications:

1. Allegra **TAB** 180 mg 1# QD **PO**.

2. Bokey EM **CAP** 100 mg 1# QD **PC** PO.

3. Concor TAB 1.25 mg 1# QD PO.

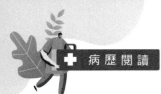
4. Fedil SR TAB 5 mg 1# QD PO.

5. Herbesser TAB 30 mg 1# **TID** AC PO.

6. Novorapid Penfill (100 U/mL 3 mL) 30# QD **SC**.

7. Pletaal TAB 50 mg 1# **BID** AC PO.

8. Atrovent+Bricanyl 1 vial **INH** BID.

9. Mubroxol TAB 30 mg 1# QID PO.

10. Unasyn **INJ** 1.5 mg **Q12H** **IV** drip.

11. IVF with N/S 500 mL QD.

12. Nosma CAP 125 mg 1# BID PO.

13. Harnalidge TAB 0.2 mg 1# BID PO.

14. Dampurine TAB 25 mg 1# QD PO.

Attending Physician: ×××

Resident: △△△

Stat Order

1. Insulin Actrapid 10U SC PRN (IF BS>350).

2. Glucose (Fasting/dextrometer) × 1 stat.

3. BUN (Blood Urea Nitrogen) × 1 stat.

4. CRP-Nephelometry × 1 stat.

5. CBC-I (WBC, RBC, Hgb, Hct, PLT) × 1 stat.

6. Creatinine × 1 stat.

7. K (Potassium) ×1 stat.

8. Na (Sodium) × 1 stat.

9. WBC differential count-LAB × 1 stat.

10. APTT (Activated partial thromboplast) × 1 stat (CM).

11. Prothombin time-LAB × 1 stat (CM).

Attending Physician: ×××

Resident: △△△

病歷小幫手

Standing Order 與 Stat Order 的區別

長期醫囑(Standing Order)

・ 常規性的治療或給藥。

・ 自開立醫囑時間起，可持續執行，直到醫囑停止為止。

臨時醫囑(Stat Order)

・ 需立即執行的治療或給藥。

・ 僅執行一次即停止。

關鍵字彙 Keywords

字　彙	原　文	中　譯
QID	L. *Quaque in diem*, four times a day	一天四次
QD	L. *quaque die*, every day	一天一次
TAB	tablet	錠劑
PO	by mouth	口服
CAP	capsule	膠囊
PC	L. *post cibum*, after meal	飯後
TID	L. *ter in die*, three times a day	一天三次
SC	subcutanous	皮下注射
BID	L. *Bis in die*, twice a day	一天兩次
INH	inhalation	吸入
INJ	injection	注射
Q12H	L. *quaque 12 hora*, every 12 hours	每 12 小時一次
IV	intravenous	靜脈注射
STAT	immediately	立即
CM	coming morning	明晨

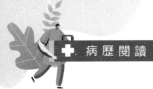

Consultation Sheet

姓名：○○○　　病歷號碼：××××××　　床號：××　　　　出生日期：****-*-*

性別：男　　　入院日期：2023-1-1　　開單科別：一般內科　　照會科別：整形外科

The 60 year-old male had a history of type 2 DM for 5 years. One chronic ulcer over his left plantar region, about 3×3 cm^2 and deep to the muscle layer, was noted. Please kindly give your expert opinion and further management. Thanks a lot.

Dr. ××× at 2023-1-2 1:00 p.m.

Reply sheet

Dear Dr. ×××,

This is a case with a diabetic ulcer over his left plantar region, stage II to III. Inflammation and discharge formation were also noted. Wound care with Iodosorb powder application is recommended at this stage. We will arrange an operation for debridement and follow up on this case afterwards. Thanks for your consultation.

Dr. ○○○ at 2023-1-2 3:00 p.m.

病歷小幫手　　　　　　　　　　　　　　　　　　　Little Helper

　　當醫師決定個案需會診其他科，請求該科醫師的專業意見時，需在會診單中註明需要照會哪一科醫師，並說明簡短的病史、身體檢查結果。被照會醫師需在醫院規定照會時間內（一般是 24 小時內）前往病人單位照會病人並填寫回覆單。一般通常會在照會單中看到的資訊會有：

1. 請求會診醫師的名字及會診理由。
2. 會診的日期與時間。
3. 檢查的發現。
4. 會診者的意見、診斷或臆斷。
5. 對診斷、治療的建議。
6. 簽章。

Discharge Summary

Internal Medicine, 60 years old, male, married, businessman.

Date of admission: 2023-1-1.

Date of discharge: 2023-1-25.

Admission Diagnosis:

1. Type 2 diabetes mellitus with poor control.

2. DM foot, left with secondary infection with sepsis.

3. HCVD.

4. URI.

5. Hyponatremia/Hyperkalemia.

6. Acute on chronic renal failure, suspected sepsis related.

7. UTI.

Discharge Diagnosis:

1. Type 2 diabetes mellitus with poor control.

2. DM foot, left with secondary infection with sepsis.

3. HCVD.

4. URI.

5. Hyponatremia/Hyperkalemia.

6. Acute on chronic renal failure, suspected sepsis related.

7. UTI.

Chief Complaint:

Shortness of breath, mild fever, with a poor healing wound on the left plantar region for months.

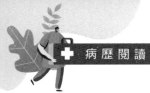

Present Illness:

This 60 year-old male patient had history of type 2 DM for 5 years with regular medical control (Novomix 38 IU BID) and OPD follow up. The latest HbA1c level was 12.2%. However, he suffered from mild fever with cough and sputum formation in the recent week. He also had the attack of urinary tract infection. Besides, he had one poor healing wound on his left plantar region, and his foot swelled in the winter. In recent 3 days, swelling, heat sensation, and redness were found on his left foot, and he felt fatigue with poor appetite, therefore, he visited our OPD this morning, where BS>500 mg/dL was noticed. He was then referred to our ER, where a series of LAB examinations disclosed leukocytosis, hyperglycemia (BS=673 mg/dL), acute on chronic renal failure, hyponatremia, mild hyperkalemia, and markedly elevated CRP level. Urine examination showed pyuria with bacteria (++). Thus, he was admitted to our ward for further management.

Brief History:

1. HCVD and Af with medical control (Urosin 1# PO QN, Fedil 1# PO QD).
2. The history of major operation: diabetic retinopathy, OS s/p OP, and cataract, OS s/p OP.

Course and Treatment:

The patient was admitted to our ward on 2023-1-1 under the impression of type 2 DM, diabetic foot with secondary infection, HCVD, UTI and URI due to shortness of breath, mild fever, and a poor healing wound on the left plantar region for months. During the hospitalization, the patient received a series of examinations and continuous RI drip was prescribed to control blood sugar, and antibiotic with Oxacillin+Unasyn were prescribed to control infection. We also consulted the PS and **CVS** specialists to evaluate his condition of his diabetic foot and the possibility of **PAOD**. Since the major circulation of his left low limb was not too bad, the CVS specialist suggested no urgent indication of surgical intervention (bypass). The PS specialist arranged surgical schedule on 2023-1-4, but it was cancelled due to atrial fibrillation around 165/min happened in **OR**. We consulted the CVS specialist and prescribed Herbesser and Concor to control his atrial fibrillation. We also adjusted the insulin to Novorapid+Lantus to keep adequate blood sugar control. Wound dressing was performed to control diabetic foot with secondary infection. Surgical intervention with **debridement** was done on 2023-1-7 and the wound condition is stable with regular topical Iodine usage thereafter. The general condition of the patient improved gradually and was then discharged on 2023-1-25 under stable condition with no other complication noted.

Review of Systems:

Throughout the whole course of present illness, the patient also suffered from symptoms mentioned as below: Chills(-), fever(+), night sweating(-), cough(+), sputum(+), hemoptysis(-), epistaxis(-), chest tightness(-), chest pain(-), SOB(+), exertional dyspnea(-), orthopnea(-), abdominal pain(-), anorexia(+), dysphagia(-), nausea(-), vomiting(-), constipation(-), diarrhea(-), hematemesis(-), hematochezia(-), melena(-), dysuria(-), oligouria(-), body weight loss(-).

1. Vital signs: BT: 37.2℃, PR: 84/min, RR: 22~24/min, BP: 148/82 mmHg.

2. Chest: Symmetrical and free expansion, breathing sound (+), bil., rhonchi.

3. Neurological: Hypoesthesia of limbs.

關鍵字彙 Keywords

字　彙	原　文	中　譯
CVS	cardiovascular surgery	心臟血管外科
PAOD	peripheral arterial occlusive disease	周邊動脈阻塞性疾病
OR	operative room	開刀房
Debridement		清創術

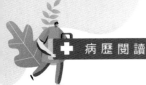
Laboratory:

1. Blood Gas Analysis

Date	pH	PCO$_2$	PO$_2$	BE	HCO$_3^-$
2023/1/1	7.333	40.6 mmHg	32.1 mmHg	−4.8 mmol/L	21.1 mmol/L

2. BCS

Date	Glucose PC	BUN	Creatinine	AST	ALK-P	Albumin	Sodium	Potassium	CRP
2023/1/1	589 mg/dL	36 mg/dL	2.1 mg/dL	10 U/L	70 U/L	3.5 g/dL	134 mEq/L	5.5 mEq/L	16 mg/dL

3. CBC

Date	WBC	RBC	Hb	Hct	MCV	PLT	Neutrophils	Monocytes	Basophils
2023/1/1	14,400 μL	4.39×10^6/μL	14 g/dL	41%	87 fL	292,000 μL	70.2%	7.5%	2.4%

4. Urine Routine

Date	Acetone	OB	Pro	Bil	S.G	pH	Nit	RBC	WBC	Bacteria
2023/1/1	1+	1+	+	−	1.019	5.0	−	20~30	>100/HPF	++

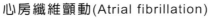

護理小幫手　　　　　　　　　　　　　　　　　　　　　Little Helper

心房纖維顫動(Atrial fibrillation)

　　為一種常見的心律不整現象，起因於心房取代了正常負責發出電信號的竇房結，導致發作時心臟會出現快速紊亂的跳動，跳動的速度可達每分鐘350~600次，可能伴隨頭暈或是呼吸短促。

Radiology & Imaging Reports:

2023-1-1 CXR:

1. Both lung parenchyma showed normal appearance without evidence of focal mass lesion.
2. Normal distribution of the pulmonary vessels was noted.
3. The heart size was within normal limit.
4. The bony structures, including bilateral ribs, scapula, clavicles and vertebral bodies, showed normal appearance without evidence of fracture.

2023-1-1 Foot, L'T X-ray:

1. Deformity, erosion and degenerative change of the left plantar region is identified.
2. Mild osteoporosis.
3. No other remarkable abnormality is seen.

Invasive Intervention Procedures:

Surgical intervention with debridement was done on 2023-1-7 and the wound condition is stable with regular iodine topical use thereafter.

Recommendations & Medications:

1. OPD F/U.
2. BD PEN Needle 31G/5 MM 1# QN EXT × 5 days.
3. Insulin Syringe 30G 0.3 c.c. 1# TID EXT × 5 days.
4. Allegra TAB 180 mg 1# QD PO × 5 days.
5. Bokey EM CAP 100 mg 1# QD PC PO × 5 days.
6. Concor TAB 1.25 mg 1# QD PO × 5 days.
7. Fedil SR TAB 5 mg 1# QD PO × 5 days.
8. Herbesser TAB 30 mg 1# TID AC PO × 5 days.
9. Novorapid Penfill 100 U/mL 3 mL 30# QD SC × 5 days.
10. Pletaal TAB 50 mg 1# BID AC PO × 5 days.

Attending Physician: ×××

Resident: △△△

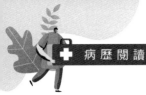
 護理小幫手 Little Helper

　　糖尿病足為糖尿病常見的併發症之一，由於血液循環改變及神經病變造成下肢敏感度、疼痛感降低，當受傷後未及時發現，易導致感染、侵犯深部組織，嚴重時會有截肢的可能。因此，糖尿病的病人應特別重視足部護理，包括：

1. 教導做下肢運動，以促進血液循環。
2. 養成每日清潔雙足，並定期修剪趾甲。
3. 選擇舒適合腳的鞋，不可以赤腳走路。
4. 吸菸會造成血液循環不佳，應戒菸。
5. 病人之冷熱感較不敏感，避免用熱水袋、小電毯、烤燈等，以防燙傷。
6. 維持血糖穩定，以防造成神經病變。

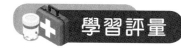

一、選擇題

( )1. 以下何者不是病人的主要住院診斷？(A)Type 2 DM　(B)HCVD　(C)URI　(D)Hypoglycemia

( )2. 請問病人的過去病史中有提及糖尿病視網膜病變，是哪一眼？(A)右眼　(B)左眼　(C)雙眼　(D)以上皆非

( )3. 病人入院時抽血液常規中，有測 PLT，中譯為何？(A)白血球數值　(B)紅血球數值　(C)血小板數值　(D)感染指數

( )4. 病人入院後，為監測血糖變化，醫囑說明測量次數為何？(A)QD/AC　(B)BID/AC　(C)TID/AC　(D)QID/AC

( )5. 請問此病人左足底區糖尿病潰瘍有會診哪科醫師協同醫療照護？(A)整形外科　(B)泌尿外科　(C)一般外科　(D)骨科

二、配合題

( )1. Hyperglycemia

( )2. Renal failure

( )3. Nephropathy

( )4. Tricuspid

( )5. Consultation

( )6. Diagnosis

( )7. Hyponatremia

( )8. Sputum

( )9. Dysphagia

( )10. Conjunctiva

(A)痰液

(B)會診

(C)心臟衰竭

(D)結膜

(E)高血鈣

(F)神經病變

(G)高血糖

(H)尿液

(I)腎臟病變

(J)吞嚥困難

(K)二尖瓣

(L)腎衰竭

(M)三尖瓣

(N)手術

(O)診斷

(P)低血糖

(Q)低血鈉

(R)說話困難

三、填充題

請寫出以下縮寫或生字之全文及中譯。

1. DM   _____

2. OPD   _____

3. ER   _____

4. SOB   _____

5. CRP   _____

6. UTI   _____

7. Impression   _____

8. Echocardiography   _____

9. Leukocytosis   _____

10. Hyperkalemia   _____

學習評量解答
請掃描 QR Code

03 | CHAPTER

外科病歷

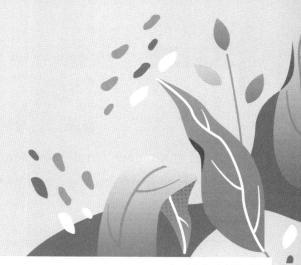

作者｜林玫君

Admission Note
Progress Note
Order Sheet
Operation Note
Operation Room Record
Consultation Sheet
Reply Sheet
Discharge Summary

☑ 閱讀導引

1. 了解病人主訴與現在病史的關係。
2. 分析現在病史與過去病史之關聯性。
3. 分析現在病史、檢驗值與治療措施的合適性。

☑ PREVIEW

閱讀本章前，請讀者先自行預習膽結石與膽囊炎相關知識喔！

1. 膽結石與膽囊炎的發生原因有哪些？常見的症狀為何？
2. 膽結石與膽囊炎常見治療為何？
3. 了解腹腔鏡膽囊切除術(laparoscopic cholecystectomy, LC)的執行過程及術後照護。

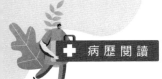

Admission Note

General surgery, male, 45 years old, Taipei, engineer.

Source of information: The patient.

Chief Complaint:

Sudden onset of **RUQ** abdominal pain since 2 days ago.

Present Illness:

According to the statement of the patient himself, he is a 45 year-old married Taiwanese male. Sudden onset of RUQ abdominal pain was noted since 2 days ago, and he came to our ER on 2023/1/2 for help, where abdominal sonogram and **CT** scan showed **gallstones** with acute **cholecystitis**. Antibiotics and **GS/GI** OPD follow up was suggested. After the inflammatory condition had become better, he was admitted to our ward for a schedule **laparoscopic cholecystectomy**.

Past History:

1. History of gout attack without medicine control 1+ years ago.
2. History with abdominal blunting injury **s/p** **Exp. Lap.** surgery due to traffic accident 10+ years ago.
3. **NKA**.

Personal History:

1. Habit of smoking: 1 **PPD** for 20+ years.
2. Habit of alcohol drinking: Social drinking.
3. The history of occupation disease: Nil.
4. The history of traveling in recent 3 months: Denied.
5. The history of drug abuse: Denied.

關鍵字彙 Keywords

字　彙	原　文	中　譯
RUQ	right upper quadrant	右上象限
CT	computed tomography	電腦斷層掃描
Gallstones		膽結石
Cholecystitis	-itis，炎	膽囊炎
GS	general surgery	一般外科
GI	gastroenterology	胃腸科
Laparoscopic cholecystectomy	lapar-，腹 -ectomy，切除術	腹腔鏡膽囊切除術
s/p	status post	在……處置之後。用來表示一個疾病後面接什麼處置
Exp. Lap.	exploratory laparotomy	剖腹探查術
NKA	no known allergy	無過敏病史
PPD	packs per day	每日（香菸）數包

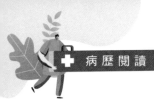

Family History:

No particular finding.

Review of Systems:

RUQ pain and a protruding mass over an old scar along the abdominal midline(+). Weight change(-), chills(-), fever(-), skin rash(-), headache(-), dizziness(-), blurred vision(-), vertigo(-), tinnitus(-), epistaxis(-), oral ulcer(-), dyspnea(-), cough(-), hemoptysis(-), chest pain (-), orthopnea(-), paroxysmal nocturnal dyspnea(-), palpitation(-), edema(-), change in appetite(-), nausea(-), vomiting(-), diarrhea(-), constipation(-), melena(-), change of bowel habit(-), jaundice(-), urgency or frequency of urination(-), hematuria(-), nocturia(-), urinary incontinence(-), joint pain(-), or stiffness of joint(-).

Physical Examinations:

1. General appearance: Fair.
2. Height: 175 cm, weight: 70 kg.
3. Vital sign: BT: 38.6℃, PR: 72/min, RR: 18/min, BP: 130/80 mmHg.
4. Skin: Senile skin turgor; multiple round scars over bilateral lower limbs.
5. HEENT: No anemic conjunctiva; no icteric sclera; no gum bleeding.
6. Neck and lymph nodes: Supple; enlarged thyroid; no palpable neck nodes; no enlarged nodes.
7. Chest and lung: Well expansion, bil.; clear breathing sound, bil.; no deformity of chest wall.
8. Heart: Regular heart beats; no murmurs; no JVE; $\underline{S}_1$(+), S_2(+), S_3(-), S_4(-); normal peripheral pulse.
9. Abdomen: Soft and ovoid in shape; mild tenderness over RUQ region; normal bowel sound. A abdomen surgical scar over midline due to perforation injury and a protruding mass lesion over middle of the scar.

10. Extremities: No deformity, free motion of joint movement.
11. Peripheral pulsation: <u>C</u> <u>B</u> <u>R</u> <u>F</u> <u>P</u> <u>PT</u> <u>DP</u>

        R't ++ ++ ++ ++ ++ ++ ++

        L't ++ ++ ++ ++ ++ ++ ++

12. Nervous system: Consciousness: Alert; mentality: Clear; pupils: <u>Isocoric</u> with LR; no impairment of motor or sensory function; no pathological reflex.

關鍵字彙 Keywords

字　彙	原　文	中　譯
S	sound	心音（S_1 表第一心音，以此類推）
C	carotid artery	頸動脈
B	brachial artery	肱動脈
R	radial artery	橈動脈
F	femoral artery	股動脈
P	popliteal artery	膝膕動脈
PT	posterial tibial artery	脛後動脈
DP	dorsalis pedis artery	足背動脈
Isocoric		瞳孔等大、對光有反應

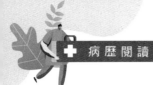
Laboratory:

1. BCS

Date	Glucose PC	BUN	Cr.	AST	ALK-P	Sodium	Potassium	Chloride	Total Bilirubin
2023/1/2	118 mg/dL	12 mg/dL	1.0 mg/dL	15 U/L	12 U/L	141 mmol/L	3.9 mmol/L	102 mmol/L	1.1 mg/dL

2. CBC

Date	WBC	RBC	Hb	Hct	MCV	PLT	Neutrophils	Lymphcytes	Monocytes
2023/1/2	11,680/uL	$4.66×10^6$/uL	14g/dL	43.3%	92.8fL	248,000/uL	76.5%	23.7%	10.3%

3. Coagulation

Date	PT P't	PT MNPT	INR	APTT P't	APTT control
2023/1/2	9.9 sec	11.0 sec	0.9	29.1 sec	29.7 sec

4. Blood type

Date	ABO RESULT	RH TYPE
2023/1/2	Blood type O	Positive

病歷小幫手

Little Helper

病歷中的 "clinical correlation" 意義為何？

　　當病人的影像學檢查發現到有某些異常，但它對病人未必是有意義的，可能也沒有造成病人的不適，此時需要再做其他更進一步的診斷性檢查，以提供醫師做診斷。例如，40 歲以上成人的脊髓 MRI 檢查可能都有些變化，但這些實際上並沒有造成不適或疾病。因此醫師會在病歷中記錄書寫 "suggest clinical correlation......" 即表示建議再做其他檢查，看看是否有顯著的發現。

Radiology & Imaging Reports:

2023-1-2 SONO. whole abdomen study

1. The liver parenchyma showed fatty infiltration.
2. The gallbladder showed small contraction and wall thickening, with small gallstones. Suggest clinical correlation to rule out chronic cholecystitis.
3. The diameter of **CBD** was measured about 0.73 cm.
4. Mild dilatation of the left lobe **IHDs** was noted.
5. A renal cyst (size: about 1.0 cm) in the lower pole of left kidney was noted.

2023-1-2 chest, P-A view

1. Suspect a small nodule in the peripheral region of right lower lung zone, recommend check CT study for further evaluation.
2. Mild scoliosis of the **T-spine** was identified.

2023-1-2 abdomen without/with contrast-C.T.

1. Mild dilatation of the both lobes IHDs is identified, but without evidence of biliary stone or soft-tissue lesion impaction. Suggest clinical correlation and check **ERCP** or **MRCP** to rule out a tiny distal CBD stone.
2. Small contraction of the gallbladder was noted.
3. Two small renal cysts about 1.3 cm in the middle and lower pole of left kidney were noted.

2023-1-3 **UGI** endoscopy

1. Esophagus: **Hiatal hernia**.
2. Mucosal breaks over **EG junction** < 5 mm, **GERD**, **LA Grade** A.
3. Stomach: Superficial gastritis, **antrum**.
4. Duodenum: Negative up to the second portion.
5. Suggestion: Medications, education and GI OPD follow-up.

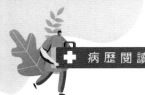

 關鍵字彙 Keywords

字　彙	原　文	中　譯
UGI	upper gastrointestinal	上腸胃道
Hiatal hernia		裂孔疝氣
EG junction	esophagogastric junction	食道胃交界處
GERD	gastroesophageal reflux disease	胃食道逆流疾病
LA Grade	LosAngeles Grade	洛杉磯分類標準分級
antrum		胃竇
CBD	common bile duct	總膽管
IHDs	intrahepatic bile ducts	肝內膽管
without/with contrast-C.T.		同一次檢查中分別照相取得無顯影劑狀態和有顯影劑狀態的兩個系列的電腦斷層影像（方便比較）
ERCP	Endoscopic retrograde cholangiopancreatography	內視鏡逆行性膽胰管造影
MRCP	magnetic resonance cholangiopancreatography	核磁共振膽管及胰臟造影
T-spine	thoracic spine	胸椎

護理小幫手

Little Helper

 食道炎的分級

食道炎的診斷分級標準為依據洛杉磯分類標準 (The LosAngeles classification)，以內視鏡依其嚴重程度分為 4 級：

1. A 級：一條或多條黏膜破損（糜爛、潰瘍）小於或等於 5 mm，並不超過兩條黏膜皺摺。
2. B 級：一條或多條黏膜破損大於 5 mm，但並不超過兩條黏膜皺摺。
3. C 級：黏膜破損在兩條黏膜皺摺間互相延續或融合，但不超過 75%的食道管腔。
4. D 級：黏膜破損在兩條黏膜皺摺間互相延續或融合，且超過 75%的食道管腔。

Impression:

1. Gallstones with cholecystitis.
2. Abdominal injury s/p operation 10+ years ago with a new-onset ventral incisional hernia.
3. GERD, LA Grade A.

Diagnostic Plans:

Check **B/R**, **E-8**, total bilirubin, PT/**PTT**, CXR, **EKG** for evaluation of pre-operative condition.

Therapeutic Plans:

1. Prophylactic antibiotics before operation.
2. Arrange operation of laparoscopic cholecystectomy and ventral incisional hernia repair.
3. Adequate pain control and wound care after surgery.

Educational plans:

Explain the indications, methods, risks and complications of the operation.

Attending Physician:×××

Resident:△△△

關鍵字彙 Keywords

字　彙	原　文	中　譯
B/R	blood routine	血液常規檢查
E-8	electrolyte-8	八項電解質
PTT	partial thromboplastin time	部分凝血酶原時間
EKG（也有人稱 ECG）	electrocardiogram	心電圖

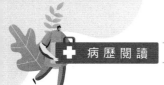

Progress Note

General surgery, male, 45 years old, Taipei, engineer.

Date of admission: 2023-01-02.

2023-1-5

#1 Acute cholecystitis, Post-op Day 1

S: Mild fever and painful sensation on surgical wounds were noted especially when walking.

O:

1. Vital signs: Stable, no high fever.

2. **J-P drain**: Clear, yellowish color, no bile noted, 40 mL in amount.

3. Abdomen: Soft, flat in shape, with decreased bowel sounds and tenderness over surgical wound sites with no rebounding pain.

A: Acute cholecystitis, status post laparoscopic cholecystectomy with surgical wound pain, in recovery status.

P:

1. Keep current empiric antibiotic and pain-killer treatment.

2. Change dressing of wound every day.

3. Closely follow up the amount and color of the drainage fluid in the J-P drain.

Attending Physician: ×××

Resident: △△△

Order Sheet

General surgery, male, 45 years old, Taipei, engineer.

Date of admission: 2023-01-02.

Pre-OP Order

2023-1-3

1. Sign the consent & permit form.

2. NPO since **MN**.

3. Check B/R, E-8, total bilirubin, PT/PTT, blood grouping, RH typing, CXR, EKG, UGI endoscopy, Abd. sono, and Abd. CT.

4. Sent P't to OR on call.

5. Set **IVF** G_5S 100 mL/hr after NPO.

6. Cefazolin 1,000 mg IV drip stat.

Attending Physician: × × ×

Resident: △△△

Post-OP Order

2023-1-4

1. Change dressing-small (<10 cm) 1 次 QD.

2. On full diet.

3. On GS routine.

4. Take vital signs QID.

5. Bain 10 mg/mL Q6H PRN **IM**.

6. Scanol 500 mg 1# QID PRN PO.

7. Cefazolin 1,000 mg IV drip Q6H×2 days.

Attending Physician: × × ×

Resident: △△△

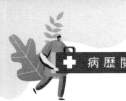

 關鍵字彙 Keywords

字　彙	原　文	中　譯
J-P drain	Jackson-Pratt drain	J-P 傷口引流管
MN	midnight	半夜、午夜
IVF	intravenous fluid	靜脈輸液
IM	intramuscular injection	肌肉注射

Thinking About

1. 個案從急診室入院後所做的檢查中有哪些異常發現證實其為膽囊炎，同時還發現個案有哪些問題？
2. 何謂手術前的預防性抗生素？經驗性抗生素？
3. 一般外科手術前準備有哪些？
4. 手術時間 On call 的意思為何？

護理小幫手

Little Helper

 腹腔鏡膽囊切除術前會在腹腔內注入二氧化碳，然後在腹部表面開 3~4 個小切口，連接套管、腹腔鏡、攝影機等。腹腔鏡深入腹腔分離總膽管及膽囊後，再將膽囊切除移出。依病情病人可能會放置傷口引流管引流。

Operation Note

Date of operation: 2023-1-4.

Preoperative Diagnosis:

1. Gallstones with cholecystitis.
2. Abdominal injury s/p operation 10+ years ago with a new-onset ventral incisional hernia.
3. GERD, LA Grade A.

Postoperative Diagnosis:

1. Gallstones with cholecystitis s/p laparascopic cholecystectomy.
2. Abdominal injury s/p operation 10+ years ago with a new-onset ventral incisional hernia s/p ventral incisional hernia repair surgery.

Operation Performed:

Laparoscopic cholecystectomy + ventral incisional hernia repair with **mesh patches**.

Surgeon: ○○○

Assistant 1: ○○○   Assistant 2: ○○○   Assistant 3: ○○○

Operation Finding:

1. A protruding mass lesion over abdominal midline of the previous incision wound, which ventral incisional hernia was impressed.
2. Severe adhesion between **omentum** to gallbladder due to previous inflammatory reaction.
3. Well dissected the cystic duct and artery and closure with **endoclips**.
4. Closure of the ventral incisional hernia with mesh.

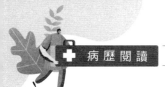

Surgical incision: <u>Subcostal</u> & <u>epiumbilical</u> incision.

Anesthesia: General.

Operation Position: Supine position.

Disinfectant: Alchohol Betadine + 75% Alchohol.

Description of Operation:

1. Under general anesthesia, the patient was put on supine position, three **<u>trocars</u>** were placed; an 10/11 mm trocar above umbilical, an additional 10/11 mm trocar at the midline, and a 5 mm trocars at the axillary line.

2. The laparoscope was inserted through the trocar. A straight locking **<u>grasper</u>** was inserted through one axillary trocar and used to apply upward traction on the gallbladder.

3. The gallbladder, still retracted by the first grasper, but was then dissected from its surrounding tissue with an additional grasper. When the cystic duct and artery had been identified, the surgeon might use the **<u>electrocautery hook</u>** to separate the tissue.

4. The cystic artery was then ligated with a **<u>titanium clamp</u>**. An additional clip was placed over the cystic duct at the base of the gallbladder.

5. The gallbladder was then removed from the liver bed with the electrocautery hook and delivered from the wound in a **<u>retrieval</u>** bag.

6. We dissected and performed lysis adhesion of the intestine by **<u>electro-coagulator</u>** and **<u>contra-release</u>** to suture the outer layer. A mesh was placed on the layer of the abdominal wall for coverage and closure of the wound.

7. The peritoneum was repaired with sutures and the wound was closed in layers after adequate irrigation and **<u>hemostasis</u>**.

8. Throughout the whole course, the procedures were done smoothly and the patient stood it well.

關鍵字彙 **Keywords**

字　彙	原　文	中　譯
Mesh patches		人工網層、疝氣修補網
Omentum		大網膜
Endoclips		止血金屬夾
Subcostal	sub-，下、次	肋下
Epiumbilical	epi-，上	肚臍上
Trocars		套管、套針
Grasper		抓握器、組織抓鉗
Electrocautery hook		電灼鉤
Titanium clamp		鈦夾
Retrieval		取回
Electro-coagulator		電燒、電凝器
Contra-release		一種可吸收的縫線
Hemostasis		止血

 Thinking About ////////////////////////////////////

1. 請問術後病程記錄中醫師開立的合宜的疼痛控制，意義為何？

2. 請問此個案術後照護重點為何？個案身上應該有哪些管路？

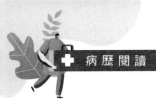
Operation Room Record

執行日期 2023 年 1 月 4 日

姓名	×××	病歷號	○○○○○○	床號	××	☑□ 門急 診診	時 段		診		號
☑男 □女	出生××年××月 ××日	科別代號		醫師代號		□ 健保	□ 自費	□ 員工	□ 員眷	□ 特約	
麻醉方式	GA	流動護士	○○○	手術開始時間：		年	月	日	時	分	
麻醉醫師	○○○	刷手護士	○○○	手術結束時間：		年	月	日	時	分	

術前診斷	Gallstones with cholecystitis.
	Abdominal injury s/p operation 10+ years ago with a new-onset ventral incisional hernia.
	GERD, LA Grade A.

臨床發現	Gallstones with cholecystitis
	Abdominal injury s/p operation 10+ years ago with a new-onset ventral incisional hernia.

術後診斷	Gallstones with cholecystitis s/p laparascopic cholecystectomy.
	Abdominal injury s/p operation 10+ years ago with a new-onset ventral incisional hernia.

手　術　名　稱	手術編號	主　刀	副　刀	點　數
1. Laparoscopic cholecystectomy + ventral incisional hernia repair with mesh patches				
2.				
3.				
4.				
5.				

失血量	minimal	病患狀況	stable	先前病理切片號碼	nil

檢體	gallblader		

分類	Small 小<5 cm 25001 件	Medium 中>5 cm 25002 件	Large 大 25003 件	超大件 25004 件	Liver biopsy 25005 件	電子顯微鏡檢查 25014 件	骨髓(Marrow) 25019 件

Operative Findings:

- Gallbladder
- Incision
- Laparoscope

1. A protruding mass lesion over abdominal midline of the previous incision wound, which ventral incisional hernia was impressed.
2. Severe adhesion between omentum to gallbladder due to previous inflammatory reaction.
3. Well dissected the cystic duct and artery and closure with endoclips.
4. Closure of the ventral incisional hernia with mesh.

醫師簽名	○○○	代　　號	

批價員		電腦編號		費用合計	

Consultation Sheet

姓名：○○○　病歷號碼：×××××　床號：××　　　　出生日期：×××××

性別：男　　入院日期：2023-1-2　　開單科別：一般外科　照會科別：眼科

The 45 year-old married male had the history of acute cholecystitis. He had a symptom of itching sensation with discharge from his right eye. Thus, we need your expertise for further evaluation and management. Thanks a lot.

Dr. ××× at 2023-1-6 10:30 a.m.

Reply Sheet

Dear Dr. ×××,

The 45 year-old married male had the history of acute cholecystitis. And the physical examination revealed redness with congestion of the right eye, acute conjunctivitis was highly suspected. Topical use of antibiotic eye drops was recommended. Thanks for your consultation.

Dr. ○○○ at 2023-1-6 4:00 p.m.

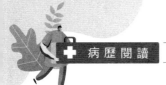

Discharge Summary

General surgery, 45 years old male, married, engineer.

Date of admission: 2023-1-2.

Date of discharge: 2023-1-10.

Admission Diagnosis:

1. Gallstones with cholecystitis.
2. Abdominal injury s/p operation 10+ years ago with a new-onset ventral incisional hernia.
3. GERD, LA Grade A.

Discharge Diagnosis:

1. Gallstones with cholecystitis s/p laparascopic cholecystectomy.
2. Abdominal injury s/p operation 10+ years ago with a new-onset ventral incisional hernia s/p ventral incisional hernia repair surgery.

Chief Complaint:

Sudden onset of RUQ abdominal pain.

Brief History:

According to the statement of the patient himself, he is a 45 year-old married Taiwanese male. Sudden onset of RUQ abdominal pain was noted since 2 days ago, and he came to our ER on 2023/1/2 for help, where abdominal sonogram and CT scan showed gallstones with acute cholecystitis. Antibiotics and GS/GI OPD follow up was suggested. After the inflammatory condition had become better, he was admitted to our ward for a schedule laparoscopic cholecystectomy.

Review of Systems:

RUQ pain and a protruding mass over an old scar along the abdominal midline(+). Weight change(-), chills(-), fever(-), skin rash(-), headache(-), dizziness(-), blurred vision(-), vertigo(-), tinnitus(-), epistaxis(-), oral ulcer(-), dyspnea(-), cough(-), hemoptysis(-), chest pain (-), orthopnea(-), paroxysmal nocturnal dyspnea(-), palpitation(-), edema(-), change in appetite(-), nausea(-), vomiting(-), diarrhea(-), · constipation(-), melena(-), change of bowel habit(-), jaundice(-), urgency or frequency of urination(-), hematuria(-), nocturia(-), urinary incontinence(-), joint pain(-), or stiffness of joint(-).

Physical Examinations:

1. General appearance: Fair.

2. Height: 175cm, weight: 70 kg.

3. Vital sign: BT: 38.6°C, PR: 72/min, RR: 18/min, BP: 130/80 mmHg.

4. Skin: Senile skin turgor; multiple round scars over bilateral lower limbs.

5. HEENT: No anemic conjunctiva; no icteric sclera; no gum bleeding.

6. Neck and lymph nodes: Supple; enlarged thyroid; no palpable neck nodes; no enlarged nodes.

7. Chest and lung: Well expansion, bil.; clear breathing sound, bil.; no deformity of chest wall.

8. Heart: Regular heart beats; no murmurs; no JVE; S_1(+), S_2(+), S_3(-), S_4(-); normal peripheral pulse.

9. Abdomen: Soft and ovoid in shape; mild tenderness over RUQ region; normal bowel sound. A abdomen surgical scar over midline due to perforation injury and a protruding mass lesion over middle of the scar.

10. Extremities: No deformity, free motion of joint movement.

11. Peripheral pulsation:　**C　B　R　F　P　PT　DP**

    R't++ ++ ++ ++ ++ ++　++

    L't ++ ++ ++ ++ ++ ++　++

12. Nervous system: Consciousness: Alert; mentality: Clear; pupils: Isocoric with LR; no impairment of motor or sensory function; no pathological reflex.

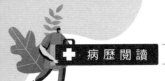

Laboratory:

1. BCS

Date	Glucose PC	BUN	Cr.	AST	ALK-P	Sodium	Potassium	Chloride	Total Bilirubin
2023/1/2	118 mg/dL	12 mg/dL	1.0 mg/dL	15U/L	12U/L	141 mmol/L	3.9 mmol/L	102 mmol/L	1.1 mg/dL

2. CBC

Date	WBC	RBC	Hb	Hct	MCV	PLT	Neutrophils	Lymphcytes	Monocytes
2023/1/2	11,680/uL	4.66×10^6/uL	14g/dL	43.3%	92.8fL	248,000/uL	76.5%	23.7%	10.3%

3. Coagulation

Date	PT P't	PT MNPT	INR	APTT P't	APTT control
2023/1/2	9.9 sec	11.0 sec	0.9	29.1 sec	29.7 sec

4. Blood type

Date	ABO RESULT	RH TYPE
2023/1/2	Blood type O	Positive

Radiology & Imaging Reports:

2023-1-2 SONO. whole abdomen study

1. The liver parechyma showed fatty infiltration.
2. The gallbladder showed small contraction and wall thickening, with small gallstones. Suggested clinical correlation to rule out chronic cholecystitis.
3. The diameter of CBD was measured about 0.73 cm.
4. Mild dilatation of the left lobe IHDs was noted.
5. A renal cyst (size: about 1.0cm) in the lower pole of left kidney was noted.

2023-1-2 chest, P-A view

1. Suspect a small nodule in the peripheral region of right lower lung zone, recommend check CT study for further evaluation.
2. Mild scoliosis of the T-spine was identified.

2023-1-2 abdomen without/with contrast-C.T.

1. Mild dilatation of the both lobes IHDs was identified, but without evidence of biliary stone or soft-tissue lesion impaction. Suggest clinical correlation and check ERCP or MRCP to rule out a tiny distal CBD stone.
2. Small contraction of the gallbladder was noted.
3. Two small renal cysts about 1.3 cm in the middle and lower pole of left kidney were noted.

2023-1-3 UGI endoscopy

1. Esophagus: Hiatal hernia.
2. Mucosal breaks over EG junction < 5 mm, GERD, LA Grade A.
3. Stomach: Superficial gastritis, antrum.
4. Duodenum: Negative up to the second portion.
5. Suggestion: Medications, education and GI OPD follow-up.

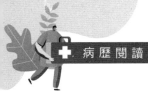

Pathological report:

Nil.

Operation Date, Method and Findings:

1. Date of operation: 2023-1-4.
2. Operation performed: Laparoscopic cholecystectomy + ventral incisional hernia repair with mesh patches.
3. Operation finding:
   (1) A protruding mass lesion over abdominal midline of the previous incision wound, which ventral incisional hernia was impressed.
   (2) Severe adhesion between omentum to gallbladder due to previous inflammatory reaction.
   (3) Well dissected the cystic duct and artery and closure with endoclips.
   (4) Closure of the ventral incisional hernia with mesh.

Course and Treatment:

The patient was admitted to our ward on 2023/1/2. During the hospitalization, the patient received a series of examinations and surgical treatment with laparoscopic cholecystectomy + ventral incisional hernia repair with mesh done on 2023/1/4. The whole procedure was smooth and the patient stood it well. The patient was discharged on 2023/1/10 under stable condition, and there were no nosocomial infection nor other complication noted. OPD follow up was advised.

Complication:

Nil.

Status on Discharge:

Stable.

Recommendations & Medications:

1. Ceflexin 500 mg 1 cap Q6H PO.
2. Depyretin 500 mg 1 tab Q12H PO.
3. Norgesic 35/450 mg 1 tab TID PO.

Attending Physician: ×××

Resident: △△△

護理小幫手

Little Helper

　　腹腔鏡膽囊切除術因術後傷口小、復原快，術後 24~48 小時便可出院，為膽囊病變最常見的治療方式。術後相關護理措施包括：

1. 術後 1~2 個月建議減少吃高油脂、高膽固醇及易產氣的食物，以避免腹脹、腹瀉等情形。
2. 若腹部有放置引流管，需保護引流管周圍皮膚，勿受膽汁外滲刺激，並維持管路通暢，下床時活動時注意避免拉扯到管路。
3. 引流管正常顏色為淡紅或淡黃色且每天量少於 50 c.c.，若有顏色改變或引流量大增時，需立即通知醫師。
4. 出院後，傷口需每天換藥、保持清潔乾燥，如果有發高燒、劇烈腹痛、黃疸、傷口出現紅腫熱痛等情形時，請病人立即回醫院診治。

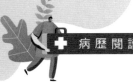

學習評量

一、選擇題

(　　)1. 請問病人入院時主訴腹痛的部位在哪？(A)左上象限　(B)右上象限　(C)左下象限　(D)右下象限

(　　)2. 請問下列何者是病患的過去病史？(A)痛風　(B)高血壓　(C)糖尿病　(D)心臟病

(　　)3. 請問病人的個人史中有提及有吸菸的習慣為何？(A)每日半包　(B)每日 1 包　(C)每日 1.5 包　(D)每日 2 包

(　　)4. 請問病人所執行的手術名稱為何？(A)膽石碎石術　(B)膽道擴張術　(C)膽囊切除術　(D)膽囊切開術

(　　)5. 請問病人所執行的手術的麻醉方式為何？(A)脊椎麻醉　(B)全身麻醉　(C)局部麻醉　(D)半身麻醉

(　　)6. 請問以下何者不是病人的出院診斷？(A)膽結石　(B)疝氣　(C)骨折　(D)胃食道逆流疾病

(　　)7. 請問病人在住院期間沒有做過的檢查為何？(A)胸部 X 光攝影　(B)腹部超音波　(C)抽血檢查　(D)痰液分析

(　　)8. 請問病人在住院期間曾會診過哪一專科？(A)胸腔科　(B)眼科　(C)腎臟科　(D)耳鼻喉科

二、配合題

1. Oral ulcer
2. Dizziness
3. Dyspnea
4. Headache
5. Epistaxis
6. Tinnitus
7. Vertigo

(A) 頭痛
(B) 頭暈
(C) 眩暈
(D) 耳鳴
(E) 鼻出血
(F) 口腔潰瘍
(G) 呼吸困難

8. Hemoptysis   (H) 咳嗽

9. Chest pain   (I) 咳血

10. Cough   (J) 胸痛

三、填充題

請寫出以下縮寫或生字之全文及中譯。

1. RUQ _____

2. cholecystectomy _____

3. cholecystitis _____

4. GS _____

5. PPD _____

6. GERD _____

7. CBD _____

8. IHDs _____

9. MRCP _____

10. ERCP _____

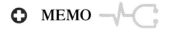

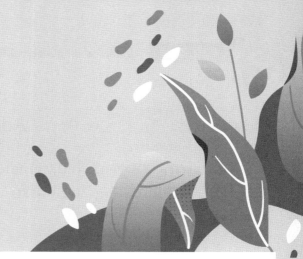

04 | CHAPTER

婦產科病歷

作者｜鄭雅敏、徐玉珍

Admission Note
Progress Note
Vaginal Delivery Note
Postpartum Note
Order Sheet
Fetal Basic US Computer Report
Consultation Sheet
Reply Sheet
Discharge Summary

☑ 閱讀導引
1. 了解病人主訴與現在病史的關係。
2. 分析現在病史與過去病史之關聯性。
3. 分析現在病史、檢驗值與治療措施的合適性。

☑ PREVIEW
閱讀本章前，請讀者先自行預習懷孕與生產相關知識喔！
1. 產前檢查的內容？
2. 懷孕的生理變化有哪些？產兆有哪些？
3. 引產的方式有哪些？
4. 產後照護注意事項。

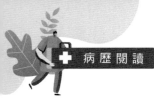
Admission Note

Obstetrics, 32 years old, female, married, housewife.

Date of admission: 2023-4-20.

Chief complaint:

Onset of **labor pain** for 1 hour.

Present illness:

This 32 year-old woman is a G_2P_1 expectant mother who is pregnant for 39 weeks. She had undergone regular prenatal visit at Dr. Lin's clinic. The results of her previous examinations, including blood sugar and blood pressure, were all normal. The screening test for Group B *Streptococcus* was negative. The basic fetal examination demonstrated normal results and no significant anomalies detected by the **ultrasonography**. She felt progressive lower abdominal pain in this morning and came to our emergency room, and then she was admitted for delivery.

OB-Gyn History:

1. Pregnancy history: G_2P_1, previous delivery: **NSD**.
2. Menstruation history:
   (1) Interval/Duration: 30 days/5~6 days.
   (2) Amount: Moderate.
   (3) **Dysmenorrhea**: Negative.
   (4) **LMP**: 2022-7-20.
   (5) **EDC**: 2023-4-27.
3. **GDM**: Nil.
   Preeclampsia: Nil.
   Gestational hypertension: Nil.
4. GBS screening: Negative.

關鍵字彙 Keywords

字　彙	原　文	中　譯
Labor pain		產痛；宮縮痛
Ultrasonography	-graphy　圖	超音波圖
OB-Gyn or OBG	obstetrics gynecology	婦產科
NSD	natural spontaneous delivery	自然生產
Dysmenorrhea	dys-　，困難、不良 meno-　，月經 -rrhea　，流量、分泌物	經痛
LMP	last menstrual period	最後一次月經
EDC	expected date of confinement	預產期
GDM	gestational diabetes mellitus	妊娠糖尿病
Preeclampsia	pre-，預、前	子癇前症
Gestational hypertension		妊娠高血壓
Goiter		甲狀腺腫大
Adventitious		外來的
Lymphadenopathy	-pathy，病變	淋巴結腫大
Paresthesia	pares-，剝	皮膚感覺異常
Os	mouthlike opening	開口
Rupture of membrane		破水
NST	non-stress test	無壓力試驗
FHB	fetal heart beat	胎兒心跳

護理小幫手 Little Helper

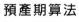 **預產期算法**
- 適用者：月經週期規則，28 天週期者。
- 算式：最後一次月經來潮之第一天的月份減 3 或加 9，日期加 7。
- 例如：最後一次月經為 8 月 12 日，則預產期為 5 月 19 日。
　　　最後一次月經為 1 月 5 日，則預產期為 10 月 12 日。

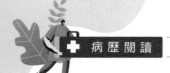
Past History:

1. Systemic diseases: Denied.

2. Operation history: Denied.

3. Current medication: Nil.

4. Allergy: Allergic to Penicillin (skin rash).

Family History:

1. Father died of complication of DM (unspecified complication).

2. Others are non-contributory.

Physical Examination:

1. Vital signs: BT: 36.5°C, PR: 85/min, RR: 14/min, BP: 130/84 mmHg.

2. General appearance: Well.
   Height: 156 cm, weight: 60 kg.

3. Consciousness: Clear, alert and oriented.

4. HEENT: Grossly normal; conjunctiva: Pinkish, not pale; sclera: Anicteric.

5. Neck: Supple, no **lymphadenopathy**, no JVE, no **goiter**.

6. Chest: Symmetric expansion and no deformity.
   Clear breath sounds, no **adventitious** breath sounds are found.

7. Heart: Regular heart beat with normal S_1 and S_2, no murmur, no S_3 and S_4 gallop.

8. Abdomen: Protruded, bowel sound: Normoactive.
   Fetal heart beat: Present.

9. Limbs: Mild edematous, peripheral pulses were all intact.

10. Neurological system: Prompt pupillary light reflex, the sensation of limbs are intact (no **paresthesia**).

Laboratory:

1. CBC

Date	RBC	Hb	MCV	MCHC	WBC	PLT	Hct
2023/4/20	$5.2×10^6/\mu L$	15.8 g/dL	96.5 fL	33.3 g/dL	8,200/μL	401,000/μL	47.4%

2. Coagulation

Date	PT	INR
2023/4/20	11.2sec	1.0

3. BCS

Date	Glucose AC	Creatinine	Albumin	Sodium	Potassium	AST	ALT	TG
2023/4/20	112 mg/dL	0.9 mg/L	4.3 g/dL	141 mEq/L	5.0 mEq/L	30 U/L	23 U/L	170 mg/L

護理小幫手　　　　　　　　　　　　　　　　Little Helper

- Glucose AC（飯前血糖）：先確定產婦是否空腹抽血。偏高者表示有糖尿病之可能性，需進一步接受葡萄糖耐受性測試才可以做正確診斷。

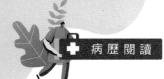
Pelvic Examination:

1. Cervix **Os**: 2 cm.

2. Station: High.

3. Effacement: Poor.

4. **Rupture of membrane**: Nil.

Non-Stress Test (NST) (figure 4-1):

1. **FHB**: Baseline: 140 bpm.

2. Variability: Reactive (130~170 bpm), without deceleration.

3. Uterine contraction: 4~5 min with power about 20~40 mmHg.

Imaging Report:

Transabdominal ultrasound revealed a placenta located in the posterior wall of the uterus and a fetus. The fetus was estimated to weight 3,145 grams.

Impression:

Pregnancy at 39 weeks with onset of labor pain.

Plan:

Prepare for normal spontaneous delivery.

Attending Physician: ×××

Resident: △△△

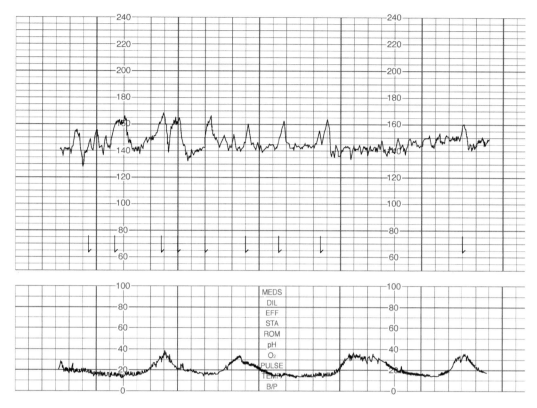

圖 4-1　無壓力試驗(NST)結果

護理小幫手

Little Helper

無壓力試驗(Non-stress test, NST)

1. 檢測對象：懷孕婦女，一般以妊娠十六週以上較容易評估。

2. 檢測目的：評估胎兒心跳狀態以及子宮收縮時胎兒心跳的變化。

3. 檢測方法：孕婦平臥於檢查檯上，裝上胎兒心跳及子宮收縮監測器，若有感覺胎動時做記號於記錄紙上，至少記錄 20 分鐘。

4. 結果判讀：20 分鐘內若至少有 2 次胎動，且伴隨每分鐘胎兒心跳增加 15 次，並持續 15 秒以上者，屬於有反應性(reactive)，為正常。若胎動過少或沒有感覺胎動，可請孕婦吃些含糖食物或飲料，也可能胎兒正在睡覺，可將腹部輕搖或用聲音振動(vibratory acoustic stimulation)來刺激胎兒，叫醒睡眠中的胎兒再記錄 20 分鐘，若還是沒有合格的胎動和胎兒心跳加速，屬於非反應性(non-reactive)，為不正常。

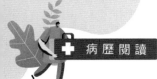

Progress Note

Obstetrics, 32 years old, female, married, housewife.

Date of admission: 2023-4-20.

2023-4-20 10:00 a.m.

#1 Labor pain

S: Labor pain: Once every 8 minutes. Severity 3/10.

O:

1. Vital signs: BT: 37.0°C, PR: 92/min, RR: 20/min, BP: 128/80 mmHg.
2. Consciousness: Clear.
3. NST: Reactive, no fetal distress.
4. Power of uterine contraction: Not effective.

A: GA 39 weeks in labor, decreased power of uterine contraction.

P:

1. Diagnostic: Pelvic examination, non-stress test, ultrasound.
2. Therapeutic: Prostagladin E_2 for induction of labor.
3. Educational: Inform the patient and family of the delivery course and complications of induction of labor.

Attending Physician: ×××

Resident: △△△

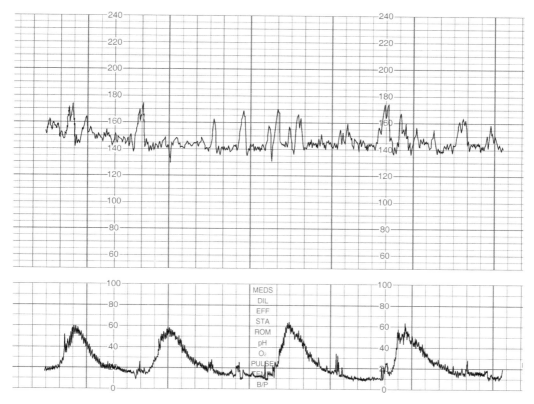

圖 4-2　胎兒心跳及子宮收縮監測圖

護理小幫手

Little Helper

　　生產時護理人員會在產婦腹部上安裝胎兒監測器，藉由圖形曲線（圖 4-2）可監視胎兒心跳速率，了解胎動時、宮縮時胎兒心跳的反應，以推測胎兒有無缺氧。監測圖的橫向格子代表時間，一格 30 秒，直向表示次數。上面一排代表胎心率的走向，下面一排代表子宮收縮時的壓力。從圖 4-2 得知目前胎兒的基礎心率約在 130~170 下／分。

　　圖 4-3 產程記錄為記錄產婦在第一產程時的狀態，包括第一列表記錄著產婦在生產過程中心跳、呼吸與血壓的變化，第二列表記錄子宮收縮的持續時間與間隔時間，第三列表格記錄胎兒心跳速率，第四列表格記錄胎兒的先露部位下降情形及子宮頸擴張程度。

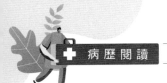

產 程 記 錄
(Progress Note of Labor)

病歷號碼：　　　　　　　姓名：　　　　　　床號：　　　　　　年齡：

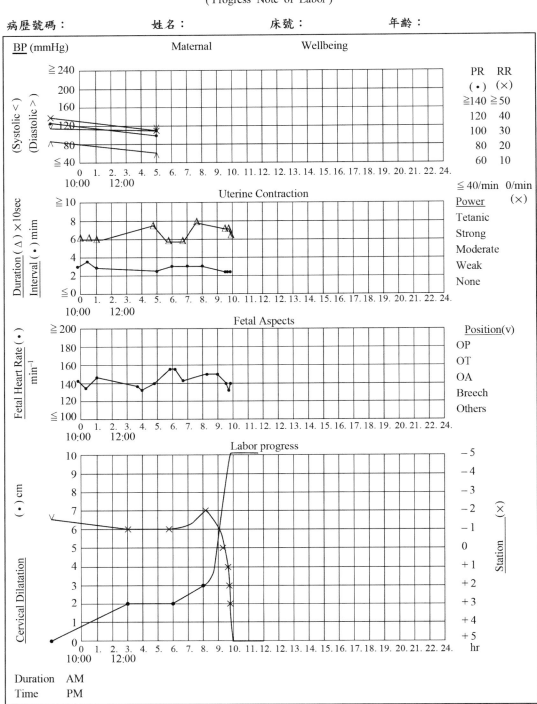

圖 4-3　產程記錄

Vaginal Delivery Note

Obstetrics, 32 years old, female, married, housewife.

Date of admission: 2023-4-20.

2023-4-20 8:00 p.m.

Under local anesthesia, median episiotomy was performed to deliver a mature, alive male baby via right occiput anterior (ROA) position.

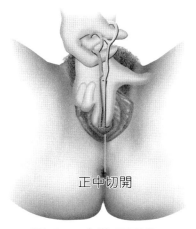

正中切開

圖 4-4　會陰切開術

Apgar score: 8→9. Newborn body weight: 3,200gm, body length: 48cm, cord around neck (1), meconium stain (1+), placenta weight: 460gm, estimated blood loss: 100mL. The median episiotomy wound was sutured with 3-0 Polysorb.

Thinking About

1. Group B *Streptococcus* 篩檢的目的為何？
2. 個案因陣痛入院時，醫師為其進行的檢查評估有哪些？有何發現？
3. 為何醫師要開立 Prostaglandin E_2 引產？

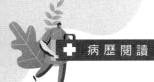
護理小幫手

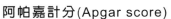

阿帕嘉計分(Apgar score)

Appearance（外觀，以膚色判斷）、Pulse（心跳）、Grimace（面部表情，抽取口鼻羊水時候，是否有哭鬧）、Activity（活動力，以肌肉張力判斷）和 Respiration（呼吸）的頭一個字母。

1. 評估時機：出生後 1 分鐘、5 分鐘時測量，如果分數過低，也就是表示狀況不好時，醫師會再記錄第 10 分鐘，甚至更後面的評估。滿分 10 分。

2. 評估項目及其計分：

分數 評估項目	2	1	0
心跳	每分鐘大於 100 下	每分鐘小於 100 下	沒有心跳
呼吸	很好，有宏亮哭聲	呼吸微弱或哭聲微弱	沒有呼吸
肌肉張力	四肢有很好的活動力	只有軟弱的彎曲	完全沒有活動
反射	抽取口鼻的羊水時，有活力的哭鬧	抽取口鼻的羊水時，只有臉部有反應	抽取口鼻的羊水時，完全沒有反應
膚色	全身通紅	軀幹紅色，四肢發紺	全身呈現缺氧黑紫

3. 結果判讀：
   - 8~10 分：是指有活力且數秒內即有宏亮的哭聲。
   - 5~7 分：代表新生兒有輕微窘迫。
   - 4 分以下：有嚴重的新生兒窘迫。因此 Apgar score 正好也可以代表新生兒在出生 1 分鐘時是否需要急救的準則。但是很明顯地，這五個徵象並不占有相同比重，其中心跳和呼吸是最重要的，而膚色相對來說是最不重要的。

Postpartum Note

Obstetrics, 32 years old, female, married, housewife.

Date of admission: 2023-4-20.

2023-4-21 9:00 a.m.

#1 <u>GA</u> 39 weeks, after vaginal delivery

S: Perineal wound pain and after pain, severity 3/10, <u>lochia</u>: Scanty

O:

1. Vital signs: BT: 36.7°C, PR: 88/min, RR: 20/min, BP: 130/78 mmHg.
2. Consciousness: Clear
3. Perineal wound: Slight <u>erythema</u>, no discharge.
4. Fundus: 1 finger below the umbilicus.

A: Normal <u>puerperal</u> recovery. Good postpartum uterine contraction.

P:

1. Diagnostic: Vital signs measurements.
2. Therapeutic: As order.
3. Educational:
   (1) Inform the patient and family about the perineal wound care and the signs of puerperal complications.
   (2) Breast-feeding educations.

Attending Physician: ×××

Resident: △△△

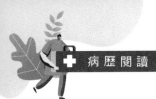

2023-4-22 9:00 a.m.

#1 GA 39 weeks, after vaginal delivery

S: Perineal wound pain and after pain, severity 2/10, lochia: Scanty.

O:

1. Vital signs: BT: 36.0°C, PR: 90/min, RR: 18/min, BP: 120/68 mmHg.
2. Consciousness: Clear.
3. Perineal wound: No discharge.
4. Fundus: 2 fingers below the umbilicus.

A: Normal puerperal recovery.

P:

1. Diagnostic: Vital signs measurements.
2. Therapeutic: **MBD** on 2023-4-22.
3. Educational:
   (1) Inform patient and family of the perineal wound care and the signs.
   (2) Breast-feeding educations.

Attending Physician: ✕✕✕

Resident: △△△

關鍵字彙 Keywords

字 彙	原 文	中 譯
GA	gestational age	妊娠週數
Lochia		惡露、產後排出物
Erythema	erythe-，紅	紅腫
Puerperal		生產的
MBD	may be discharged	允許出院

Order Sheet

Obstetrics, 32 years old, female, married, housewife.

Date of admission: 2023-4-20.

Standing Order

2023-4-20

1. Admitted under the service of Dr. Lin.

2. Diagnosis: Pregnancy at 39 weeks in labor.

3. Condition: Stable.

4. Activity: As tolerance.

5. Vital sign: QID.

6. Allergy: Penicillin.

7. Nursing: Non-stress test, doppler for fetal heart beats Q8H & PRN.

8. Diet: Prenatal diet 2,500 cal/day.

9. IV: $D_{2.5}S$ keep line.

10. Medication: Prostaglandin E_2 500 mg vaginal tablet 1/2# Q6H PRN.

11. Laboratory: Check CBC, D/C, Biochem (Glucose AC, BUN, Creatinine, AST, ALT, Albumin, Sodium, TG, Potassium), PT/PTT, U/A.

12. Obstetric sonography.

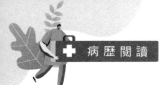

Fetal Basic US Computer Report

姓名：○○○　　　性別：女　　　出生日期：****-*-**　　病歷號碼：××××××

入院日期：2023-4-20　科別：婦產科　床號：××　　　檢查日期：2023-4-20

I. US Data

Fetal No.: 1

Position: 1 (1.**Vx** 2.**BR** 3.**TR**)

BPD: 9.2 cm　　**OFD**: 11.5 cm

AD 1: 11.0 cm

AD 2: 10.5 cm

FL: 7.5 cm

Placenta Location: 2 (1.**A** 2.**P** 3.**R** 4.**L** 5.**F** 6.**Previa**)

Grade: 3

Amniotic Fluid Index: 11.6

II. Computed Data

Gestational age: 39.0W

EDC: 2023/04/27

HC: 32.5 cm

AC: 34.5 cm

EBW: 3,145 gm

III. US Age

BPD age: 38.0W US age: 38.5W

AC age: 39.0W　**UA-MA**: 0.5W

FL: 39.5W

IV. Fetal Growth Assessment: 1

(1.**AGA**　2.**R/O SGA**　3.R/O **LGA**)

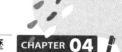

 關鍵字彙 Keywords

字　彙	原　文	中　譯
US	ultrasound	超音波
Vx	vertex	頭位
BR	breech	臀位
TR	transverse	橫位
BPD	biparietal distance	雙頂間徑
OFD	occipital-frontal distance	枕額徑
AD	abdominal distance	腹腔橫徑
FL	femur length	大腿骨長度
A	anterior	前
P	posterior	後
R	right	右
L	left	左
F	fundus	宮底
Previa		前置胎盤
HC	head circumference	頭圍
AC	abdominal circumference	腹圍
EBW	estimated body weight	預估體重
UA-MA	ultrasound age-maternal age	超音波預估胎兒年齡與根據母親月經估算胎兒年齡之差別
AGA	average for gestational age	胎兒體重適中
R/O（也有人寫作 r/o）	rule out	疑似、不排除*
SGA	small for gestational age	胎兒體重過輕
LGA	large for gestational age	胎兒體重過重

註：r/o 其實是很有趣的一個詞彙。他的原意是 rule out（排除），代表不可能。但是在台灣常常會看到病歷寫說 fever, should r/o UTI related，意思是導致發燒的原因中，UTI 是應該「最優先」被排除的那個原因，但此刻還沒被排除，而因為我們需最優先排除他才考慮其他原因，所以反而是最可能的第一診斷。所以若是把 should 或 need to 接在 r/o 前面，則此時 should r/o 表示「不能排除的意思」，也就是疑似、不排除的意思。而現今的狀況是很多人連 should 或 need to 都懶得打出來了，只單用一個 r/o 就來表示疑似的意思。

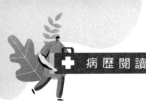

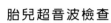 護理小幫手

Little Helper

 胎兒超音波檢查

1. 檢查目的：利用超音波測量胎兒的頭圍、腹圍，套入計算公式，預估胎兒體重。

2. 檢查項目及其意義：超音波檢查並無輻射線，它是利用聲波原理呈現影像。胎兒超音波檢查可以預估胎兒體重，評估胎兒生長是否適當，是否有過重或過輕（生長遲滯現象），此外還可以評估胎兒體內器官是否有結構上異常。胎盤、臍帶、羊水的結構皆可以利用超音波做評估。胎兒超音波檢查是現代孕婦產前檢查不可或缺的檢查項目之一。

Thinking About

1. 醫師施行會陰切開術的目的為何？
2. 自然產後記錄的重點為何？

關鍵字彙 Keyword

字　彙	原　文	中　譯
Eruption		出疹
Erythematous	erythema-，紅斑	紅斑的
Papule		丘疹
Pigmentation		著色，色素沉著
Pruritic		搔癢的
Purpura		紫斑

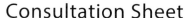

Consultation Sheet

姓名：○○○　　　　性別：女　　　　出生日期：****-*-**　病歷號碼：××××××

入院日期：2023-4-20　床號：××　　開單科別：婦產科　　照會科別：皮膚科

Clinical Diagnosis: Pregnancy 39 weeks s/p vaginal delivery.

Purpose of Consultation: For the evaluation of skin <u>eruption</u> over bilateral lower extremities.

Brief History:

This 32 year-old female patient is a pregnant woman who just delivered a male baby on 2023-4-20. She had suffered from an <u>erythematous papule</u> over bilateral lower extremities since the third trimester. It would accompany with itching and skin <u>pigmentation</u>. The symptoms became more severe in recent days. Your expertise is highly appreciated.

Dr. ××× at 2023-4-21 1:00 p.m.

Reply Sheet

Diagnosis: Pregnancy related <u>pruritic purpura</u>.

Physical Examination:

This patient was evaluated clearly. There are multiple pigmented papule, about 0.3~0.5 cm over bilateral lower extremities. She just delivered a male baby and the symptom occurred during the third trimester. The diagnosis of pregnancy related pruritic purpura would be done. It is associated with the maternal reaction to fetal testosterone. The skin eruption will resolve gradually postpartum spontaneously. I had explained the condition to patient. Topical steroid cream will help to relief the clinical symptoms. Thanks for consultation.

Dr. ○○○ at 2023-4-21 3:00 p.m.

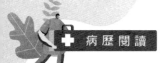

Discharge Summary

Obstetrics, 32 years old, female, married, housewife.

Date of admission: 2023-4-20.

Date of discharge: 2023-4-22.

Admission Diagnosis:

Pregnancy at 39 weeks with onset of labor pain.

Discharge Diagnosis:

1. Pregnancy at 39 weeks with labor pain s/p vaginal delivery.

2. Pregnancy related pruritic purpura.

Chief Complaint:

Onset of labor pain for 1 hour.

Brief History:

This 32 year-old woman is a G_2P_1 expectant mother who is pregnant for 39 weeks. She had undergone regular prenatal visit at Dr. Lin's clinic. The results of her previous examinations, including blood sugar and blood pressure, were all normal. The screening test for Group B *Streptococcus* was negative. The basic fetal examination demonstrated normal results and no significant anomalies detected by the ultrasonography. She felt progressive lower abdominal pain in this morning and came to our emergency room, and then she was admitted for delivery.

Past History:

1. Systemic diseases: Denied.

2. Operation history: Denied.

3. Current medication: Nil.

4. Allergy: Allergic to Penicillin (skin rash).

Physical Examination:

1. Vital signs: BT: 36.5℃, PR: 85/min, RR: 14/min, BP: 130/84 mmHg.
2. General appearance: Well.

   Height: 156 cm, weight: 60 kg.
3. Consciousness: Clear; alert and oriented.
4. HEENT: Grossly normal; conjunctiva: Pinkish, not pale; sclera: Anicteric.
5. Neck: Supple, no lymphadenopathy, no JVE, no goiter.
6. Chest: Symmetric expansion and no deformity.

   Clear breath sounds, no adventitious breath sounds are found.
7. Heart: Regular heart beat with normal S_1 and S_2, no murmur, no S_3 gallop.
8. Abdomen: Protruded, bowel sound: Normoactive. Fetal heart beat: Present.
9. Limbs: Mild edematous, peripheral pulses were all intact.
10. Neurological system: Prompt pupillary light reflex, the sensation of limbs are intact (no paresthesia).

Pelvic Examination:

1. Cervix Os: 2 cm.
2. Station: High.
3. Effacement: Poor.
4. Rupture of membrane: Nil.

Surgical Date and Method:

Vaginal delivery male baby on 2023-4-20 08:00 p.m.

Course and Treatment:

After admission, the labor course progressed gradually and she delivered a male baby transvaginally at 2023-4-20 08:00 p.m.. Median episiotomy and suture with 3-0 Polysorb continuously. Estimated blood loss was 100 mL. There was no significant postpartum complication noted and she was discharged on 2023-4-22.

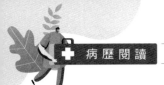

Complication:

Nil.

Laboratory:

1. CBC

Date	RBC	Hb	MCV	MCHC	WBC	PLT	Hct
2023/4/20	$5.2 \times 10^6/\mu L$	15.8 g/dL	96.5 fL	33.3 g/dL	8,200/μL	401,000/μL	47.4%

2. coagulation

Date	PT	INR
2023/4/20	11.2 sec	1.0

3. BCS

Date	Glucose AC	Creatinine	Albumin	Sodium	Potassium	AST	ALT	TG
2023/4/20	112 mg/dL	0.9 mg/L	4.3 g/dL	141 mEq/L	5.0 mEq/L	30U/L	23 U/L	170 mg/L

Radiology Report:

Nil.

Pathological Report:

Nil.

Discharge Planning:

1. Discharge condition: Stable and OPD follow up on 2023-6-10.

2. Medication: Magnesium Oxide 250 mg/tab, 1# QID PO.

Attending Physician: ×××

Resident: △△△

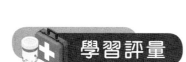學習評量

一、選擇題

(　)1. G.P.A.意指： (1)孕次 (2)活產 (3)死產 (4)流產 (5)剖腹，以上正確說明為何？(A)(2)(3)(5)　(B)(2)(3)(4)　(C)(1)(2)(4)　(D)(2)(4)(5)

(　)2. 張太太懷孕三十八週，因子宮規則收縮入院待產，詢問她的妊娠史為：生過三胎，第一胎在懷孕四週時人工流產，第二胎是雙胞胎，第三胎是男嬰，請問 GPA 寫法為？(A)$G_4P_2A_1$　(B)$G_3P_2A_1$　(C)$G_5P_3A_1$　(D)$G_4P_3A_1$

(　)3. 楊太太月經約兩週沒來，至門診求治發現已懷孕六週，表示月經規則且最後一次月經 111 年 11 月 1 日，預產期為？(A)112 年 7 月 9 日　(B)112 年 8 月 8 日　(C)112 年 9 月 10 日　(D)112 年 8 月 1 日

(　)4. 最後一次月經(LMP)，意指月經週期的哪一天？(A)第 2 天　(B)第 7 天　(C)第 5 天　(D)第 1 天

(　)5. 胎兒基礎心跳在無壓力試驗下，應介於多少 bpm？(A)100~140　(B)150~200　(C)130~170　(D)160~210

二、配合題

(　)1. Vaginal delivery

(　)2. Ultrasonography

(　)3. Preeclampsia

(　)4. Dysmenorrhea

(　)5. ROA

(　)6. Paresthesia

(　)7. GDM

(　)8. Lymphadenopathy

(　)9. Pigmentation

(　)10. $G_4P_1A_2$

(A)X 光攝影
(B)妊娠高血壓
(C)牙痛
(D)子癇症
(E)剖腹生產
(F)右枕橫位
(G)右枕前位
(H)超音波圖
(I)色素沉著
(J)經陰道自然生產

(K)感覺遲緩
(L)感覺異常
(M)妊娠糖尿病
(N)子癇前症
(O)淋巴結病變
(P)淋巴球病變
(Q)經痛
(R)懷孕四次，活產二次，流產一次
(S)懷孕四次，活產一次，流產二次

三、填充題

請寫出以下縮寫或生字之全文及中譯。

1.　預產期　_____

2.　胎兒心跳　_____

3.　破水　_____

4.　正中會陰切開術　_____

5.　惡露　_____

6.　LMP　_____

7.　MBD　_____

8.　NST　_____

9.　GBS　_____

10.　G.P.A.　_____

學習評量解答
請掃描 QR Code

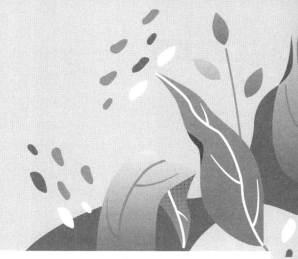

Admission Note

Progression Note

Order Sheet

Operation note

Discharge Summary

☑ 閱讀導引

1. 了解病童的主訴及病史內容。

2. 分析現在病史與過去病史之關聯性。

3. 明白病童的健康問題與醫療處置間的相關性。

4. 分析現在病史、檢驗值與治療措施的合適性。

☑ PREVIEW

閱讀本章前，請讀者先自行預習移植後淋巴異常增生疾病(PTLD)相關知識喔！

1. 兒科病歷的記錄重點為何？

2. PTLD 的發生原因與相關治療。

3. 何謂 Port-A？

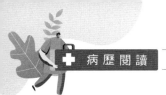

Admission Note

Pediatrics, 3 years old, female, residency: Hsinchu.

Source of information: The patient's parents.

Date of admission: 2023-1-12.

Chief Complaint:

Admitted for B-cell type **post-transplantation lymphoproliferative** disease and **Port-A catheter** removal.

Present Illness:

This 3 year-old girl has suffered from continued jaundice since she was born. **MRCP**, **HIDA scan** and liver needle **biopsy** confirmed the diagnosis of biliary atresia. **Kasai operation** was performed while she was 37 days old. The serum bilirubin level didn't reduce after the operation. She received liver transplantation seven months later. Post-transplantation biopsy revealed only mild rejection and preservation injury. The serum level of bilirubin also decreased after transplantation.

Five months later, she was admitted owing to acute **gastroenteritis**. Esophagogastroduodenogram (**EGD**) revealed multiple erythematous, ulcerative lesions in her stomach. Biopsy showed post-transplantation lymphoproliferative disease (**PTLD**) with a B cell-predominant feature. CT scan exhibited enlargement of para-aortic lymph nodes. **PET scan** confirmed the lesions located at stomach, colon and abdominal lymph nodes. Bone marrow aspiration and biopsy revealed no involvement of PTLD.

She then received **CHOP chemotherapy** initially. Then we added anti-CD20 antibody into the regimen. In addition, Ganciclovir was also given to eradicate **EBV**, which is highly correlated with the development of PTLD. The lesions gradually disappeared from the image taken by CT scan after a three-month therapeutic duration. Now she is 3 years old and

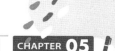

the Port-A catheter inserted has not been used for a long time. This time, she was admitted for another survey to PTLD and to receive an operation removing the Port-A catheter.

關鍵字彙 Keywords

字　彙	原　文	中　譯
Post-transplantation	post-，後 trans-，經、穿、過	移植後
Lymphoproliferative	lympho-，淋巴 -proliferative，增殖、增生	淋巴增生
Port-A catheter		人工血管
MRCP	magnetic resonance cholangiopancreatography	核磁共振膽管及胰臟造影
HIDA scan	hepatobiliary iminodiacetic acid scan or cholescintigraphy	核子醫學膽道攝影
Biopsy		組織切片檢查
Kasai operation		葛西手術
Gastroenteritis	gastr-，胃 -itis，炎	腸胃炎
EGD	esophagogastroduodenogram	上消化道內視鏡（食道、胃、十二指腸）
PTLD	post-transplantation lymphoproliferative disease	移植後淋巴異常增生疾病
PET scan	positron emission tomography scan	正子造影掃描
CHOP chemotherapy	include Cyclophosphamide, Hydroxydaunomycin, Oncovin and Prednisone	CHOP 化學治療（雞尾酒療法的一種）
EBV	Epstein-Barr virus	EB 病毒

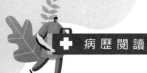

 病歷小幫手　　　　　　　　　　　　　　　　　　Little Helper

兒科病歷的記錄書寫

　　兒科病人因不同階段的個體發展，疾病種類也具有很大的差異，因此在收集病史與書寫病歷時的重點也有所不同。兒科病人病史詢問多需經由家屬或照顧者提供，以及臨床醫師的觀察，因此病歷上應註明提供資訊的來源為何。

　　兒科病人對於生長及發育的評估、預防保健、飲食狀況、遺傳性疾病及先天性異常都是詢問重點。新生兒及嬰幼兒還需要注意母親懷孕史、病史及生產史，而新生兒成熟度及身體檢查更是新生兒及早產兒照顧上重要之參考資料。

 護理小幫手　　　　　　　　　　　　　　　　　　Little Helper

Kasai Operation

　　1957 年，日本東北大學的葛西森夫教授完成世界首例的膽道閉鎖手術，因此被命名為葛西手術(Kasai Operation)。該項手術包括了三大部分：

1. 肝門纖維塊的剝離。
2. 空腸的迴路手術：在 Treitz 韌帶下 15 公分切斷空腸，取 40~60 公分做膽道通路，再將空腸做端側吻合術。
3. 將空腸接至肝門。

Past History:

1. Birth history: $G_2P_1A_1$, NSD, GA: 40 wks, BBW: 2,700 gm, **PROM** (-), neonatal jaundice (+).

2. Feeding: Full diet.

3. Vaccination: **HBV** × 3, (**DTaP-Hib-IPV**) × 3.

4. Growth and development:
   (1) BW: 14 kg (25~50 percentile).
   (2) BL: 94 cm (10~25 percentile).

5. Developmental milestone: **WNL**.

6. Maternal history:
   (1) Denied systemic disease.
   (2) No radiation or drugs exposure during pregnancy.

7. Past history:
   (1) 33 d/o: Diagnosed biliary atresia (present with prolong jaundice).
   (2) 37 d/o: s/p Kasai operation.
   (3) 7 m/o: s/p living related liver transplantation.
   (4) 12 m/o:
      • **EGD** showed multiple erythematous, ulcerative lesions.
      • Biopsy revealed B cell type post-transplantation lymphoproliferative disease.
      • EBV viral load (2904 copies/ug DNA).
   (5) 12 m/o: Chemotherapy, low dose CHOP.
   (6) 13 m/o, 14 m/o, 15 m/o: Anti-CD20 monoclonal antibody therapy.
   (7) 16 m/o: EGD showed solitary ulcerative lesions without PTLD lesions.
   (8) 22 m/o: EGD showed no organic lesion, EBV (432 copies/ug DNA).

8. No known drug or food allergy.

9. Medication: Cyclosporine A (100 mg/mL) 0.1 mL BID PO.

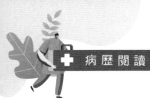

關鍵字彙 Keywords

字 彙	原 文	中 譯
PROM	premature rupture of membrane	早期破水
HBV	hepatitis B virus	B 型肝炎
DTaP-Hib-IPV	diphtheria and tetanus toxoid with acellular pertussis, inactivated polio and *haemophilus influenzae* type b vaccine	五合一疫苗（白喉、破傷風、非細胞性百日咳、b 型嗜血桿菌及不活化小兒麻痺混合疫苗）
WNL	within normal limits	在正常範圍內
EGD	esophagogastroduodenoscopy	上消化道內視鏡（食道、胃、十二指腸）

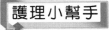 護理小幫手

Little Helper

Port-A catheter

　　Port-A (a portal and a catheter)俗稱人工血管，主要構造有一個注射入口和一條導管，經由手術方式將注射區植入鎖骨下胸腔壁的皮下，使導管經由上腔靜脈通到右心房上方，外觀看起來就像硬幣般突起。主要目的可以用來做靜脈注射、化學治療或抽血，使病人免除反覆扎針的不適。

Family History:

Non-contributory.

Physical Examination:

1. General appearance: Fair, conscious: Clear.
2. Vital signs: BT: 36.3°C, PR: 92/min, RR: 21/min, BP: 130/62 mmHg.
3. HEENT: Grossly normal.
   (1) Conjunctivae: Not pale.
   (2) Sclera: Anicteric.
   (3) Pupils: Isocoria, prompt and symmetric pupillary light reflex.
   (4) Throat: Mild injected.
4. Neck: Supple, no JVE, no **LAP**.
5. Heart: **RHB** without murmur.
6. Chest: Symmetric expansion, clear breath sounds, no crackles or wheeze.
7. Abdomen: Soft, flat, normoactive bowel sound, operation scar. Liver: 2 cm below **RCM**, spleen: Impalpable.
8. Extremities: Freely movable, no petechiae or ecchymosis.

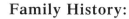

關鍵字彙 Keywords

字　彙	原　文	中　譯
LAP	Lymphadenopathy	淋巴結腫大
RHB	regular heart beat	規則心跳
RCM	Right costal margin	右側肋骨下緣

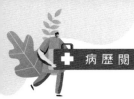
Laboratory:

1. CBC

Date	RBC	WBC	Hb	PLT	MCV	Hct	MCHC	MCH
2023/1/12	4.48×10^6/uL	5,600/uL	12.4 g/dL	176,000/uL	82.4 fL	36.4%	34.3 g/dL	28.3 pg

2. Differential count

Date	Neutrophils	Lymphocytes	Band form	Eosinophils	Monocytes	Basophils
2023/1/12	35.5%	55%	0%	0.2%	8.9%	0.2%

3. Coagulation

Date	PT	INR
2023/1/12	11 sec	0.99

4. BCS

Date	Glucose PC	BUN	Creatinine	Albumin	AST	ALT	ALP
2023/1/12	110 mg/dL	10 mg/dL	0.5 mg/L	4.68 g/dL	43 U/L	22 U/L	508 U/L
	LDH	GGT	T-/D-bilirubin	Sodium	Potassium	Cyclosporine (C2)	EBV viral load
	800 U/L	9 U/L	0.43/0.1 mg/dL	138 mEq/L	4.0 mEq/L	52.12 ng/mL	negative

Thinking About

1. 從個案的過去病史得知 PTLD 的治療過程為何？
2. 為何個案要驗 EBV、Cyclosporine？
3. 為何個案要移除 Port-A？
4. 移除 Port-A 的術前準備、術後護理為何？

Radiology & Image Reports:

1. EGD:
   (1) No visible lesions in esophagus.
   (2) Patchy **hyperemia** at the body of stomach without any visible lesions.
   (3) No visible lesions in duodenum.
      Diagnosis: **Superficial gastritis**.

2. CT scan: CT study of the abdomen before and after the use of contrast medium shows:
   (1) No evident dilatation of **intrahepatic** bile ducts.
   (2) Patent enhancement of the transplanted portal vein.
   (3) No evident abdominal fluid accumulation.
   (4) No evident enlargement of abdominal lymph nodes.

Diagnosis:

1. Biliary atresia, s/p Kasai operation and liver transplantation.
2. B cell type PTLD, s/p CHOP & anti-CD20 therapy, with disease remission.

Attending Physician: ×××

Resident: △△△

關鍵字彙 Keywords

字　彙	原　文	中　譯
Hyperemia	hyper-，過、多 -emia，血液疾病	充血
Syperficial	super-，上	表淺性
Gastritis	gastr-，胃 -itis，炎	胃炎
Intrahepatic	intra-，內、間 -hepat，肝	肝內

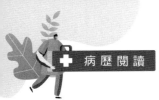

Progression Note

Pediatrics, 3 years old, female, residency: Hsinchu.

Source of information: The patient's parents.

Date of admission: 2023-1-12.

2023-1-14

#1 <u>Postoperative</u> first day

S: Pain over the wound and dry mouth. No flatus passage.

O: Dry skin and mouth. Clean dressing on the wound. Increased pulse & respiratory rate and BT (37.8°C), clear breathing sounds. Mildly distended abdomen with **<u>hypoactive</u>** bowel sounds.

A:

1. Postoperative wound pain.
2. **<u>Inadequate</u>** fluid supply.
3. Not yet recovery of normal bowel activity.

P:

1. Pain control with **<u>narcotic analgesics</u>**.
2. Increase parenteral fluid supply.
3. Menthol oil application to the **<u>periumbilical</u>** area.

2023-1-14

＃2 May be discharge

S: Less wound pain.

O:

1. Vital sign: BT: 36.6°C, PR: 78/min, RR: 16/min, BP: 125/80 mmHg.
2. Conscious: Clear.
3. Conjunctiva: Pink.
4. Chest: Symmetric.
5. BS: Clear.
6. OP wound dressing: Clear, no blood coating on gauze.
7. Hemoglobin level: 10.2 g/dL.

A: Post-OP first days.

P:

1. Wound dressing change.
2. May be discharge and OPD follow up.

Attending Physician: ×××

Resident: △△△

關鍵字彙 Keywords

字　彙	原　文	中　譯
Postoperative	post-，後	手術後
Hypoactive	hypo-，少、低	活動過少
Inadequate	in-，不	不適當
Narcotic analgesics		麻醉性止痛劑
Periumbilical	peri-，周圍	臍周圍

Order Sheet

Pediatrics, 3 years old, female, residency: Hsinchu.

Source of information: The patient's parents.

Date of admission: 2023-1-12.

Standing Order

2023-1-12

Diagnosis:

1. Biliary atresia, s/p Kasai operation and liver transplantation.

2. B cell type PTLD, s/p CHOP & anti-CD20 therapy, disease remission.

On General Pediatric routine.

Vital sign Q4H.

On full diet.

Stat Order

1. Check CBC, Creatinine, BUN, CRP, S-GOT (AST), S-GPT (ALT).

2. Urine routine examination.

3. EKG (Electrocardiography).

4. Chest X-ray (PA).

Pre-op Order (Ped)

1. Skin preparation.

2. Sign operative and anesthetic consent forms.

3. Sent patient to OR on call.

4. Cephalexin 250 gm INJ stat for sent to operating room.

5. Normal saline 500 mL INJ for antibiotic use.

Standing Order

2023-1-13 OP day

1. NAKO No.2 INJ (500 mL) run 40 mL/hr QD IV.

2. Pantogen INJ (500 mL) run 40 mL/hr QD IV.

3. Penicillin 1,200 thousands U IVD Q6H.

4. If BT>38°C Panadol (500 mg) 1/4# Q6H PRN.

5. If BT>38.5°C Purfen (400 mg) 1/4# Q6H PRN.

6. If BT>39°C Voren supp (12.5 mg) 2/3# Q6H PRN.

Stat Order

2023-1-14 post-OP day 1

1. Dressing change.

2. MBD.

3. Discharge from removing Port-A catheter.

護理小幫手

Little Helper

認識單株抗體治療

　　單株抗體治療是將藥物連接在單株抗體上，利用單株抗體的專一性將藥物帶至目標細胞。例如：將可以殺死癌細胞的藥物與對癌細胞有特異性之單株抗體結合一起，再將此結合物打入病人體內，此時，單株抗體就會把藥物帶到癌細胞處，再發揮藥效將癌細胞殺死，並且不會影響到人體正常細胞。

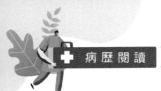

Operation note

Date of operation: 2023/1/13.

Preoperative Diagnosis:

1. Biliary atresia, s/p Kasai operation and liver transplantation.

2. B cell type PTLD, s/p CHOP & anti-CD20 therapy, disease remission.

Postoperative Diagnosis:

1. Biliary atresia, s/p Kasai operation and liver transplantation.

2. B cell type PTLD, s/p CHOP & anti-CD20 therapy, disease remission.

Operation performed: Remove a Port-A catheter.

Surgeon: ×××.

Assistant: None.

Anesthesia: <u>LA</u>-local 0.25% Marcaine.

Anesthesiologist: ○○○.

Estimated blood loss: Minimal.

Blood transfused: None.

Drains: None.

Specimens: None.

Description of Operation:

With the patient in the main operating room under adequate IV sedation and carefully monitored by anesthesia, Kefzol was given at the **time of induction.** A small towel was placed in the **intrascapular** area. The entire upper chest, on both sides, including the neck and shoulder area were **prepped** with Iodoform and draped in the usual sterile fashion. The patient was placed in a supine position and anesthetized using 0.25% Marcaine. Then, the Port-A catheter was removed and the wound was closed. The small incisions were approximated using #3-0 Vicryl suture. Then a sterile dressing was applied to the wound.

The estimate of blood loss was minimal. No transfusion was required. No drains were placed. Sponge and instrument counts were corrected at the end of the case. The patient subsequently tolerated the procedure well and was then returned to her room in a stable condition.

關鍵字彙 Keywords

字　彙	原　文	中　譯
LA	local anesthesia	局部麻醉
Time of induction		麻醉引導期
Intrascapular	intra-，內	肩胛內側
Prepped	prep	準備好

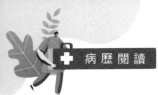

Discharge Summary

Pediatrics, 3 years old, Female, residency: Hsinchu.

Source of information: The patient's parents.

Date of admission: 2023-1-12.

Date of discharge: 2023-1-14.

Admission Diagnosis:

1. Biliary atresia, s/p Kasai operation and liver transplantation.
2. B cell type PTLD, s/p CHOP & anti-CD20 therapy, with disease remission.

Discharge Diagnosis:

1. Biliary atresia, s/p Kasai operation and liver transplantation.
2. B cell type PTLD, s/p CHOP & anti-CD20 therapy, s/p Port-A removal on 2023/01/13, with disease remission.

Chief Complaint:

Admitted for B-cell type post-transplantation lymphoproliferative disease study and Port-A catheter removal.

Brief History:

This 3 year-old girl has suffered from continued jaundice since she was born. MRCP, HIDA scan and liver needle biopsy confirmed the diagnosis of biliary atresia. Kasai operation was performed while she was 37 days old. The serum bilirubin level didn't reduce after the operation. She received liver transplantation seven months later. Post-transplantation biopsy revealed only mild rejection and preservation injury. The serum level of bilirubin also decreased after transplantation.

Five months later, she was admitted owing to acute gastroenteritis. Esophagogastroduodenogram (EGD) revealed multiple erythematous, ulcerative lesions in her stomach. Biopsy showed post-transplantation lymphoproliferative disease (PTLD) with a B cell-predominant feature. CT scan exhibited enlargement of para-aortic lymph nodes. PET scan confirmed the lesions located at stomach, colon and abdominal lymph nodes. Bone marrow aspiration and biopsy revealed no involvement of PTLD.

She then received CHOP chemotherapy initially. Then we added anti-CD20 antibody into the regimen. In addition, Ganciclovir was also given to eradicate EBV, which is highly correlated with the development of PTLD. The lesions gradually disappeared from the image taken by CT scan after a three-month therapeutic duration. Now she is 3 years old and the Port-A catheter inserted has not been used for a long time. This time, she was admitted for another survey to PTLD and to receive an operation removing the Port-A catheter.

Physical Examination:

1. General appearance: Fair, conscious: Clear.
2. Vital signs: BT: 36.3°C, PR: 92/min, RR: 21/min, BP: 130/62 mmHg.
3. HEENT: Grossly normal.
   (1) Conjunctivae: Not pale.
   (2) Sclera: Anicteric.
   (3) Pupils: Isocoria, prompt and symmetric pupillary light reflex.
   (4) Throat: Mild injected.
4. Neck: Supple, no JVE, no LAP.
5. Heart: RHB without murmur.
6. Chest: Symmetric expansion, clear breath sounds, no crackles or wheeze.
7. Abdomen: Soft, flat, normoactive bowel sound. Liver: 2 cm below RCM, spleen: Impalpable.
8. Operation scar on the abdomen.
9. Extremities: Freely movable, no petechiae or ecchymosis.

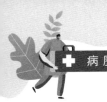

Laboratory:

Item \ Date	2023/1/12	2023/1/14
WBC	5,600/uL	
RBC	4.48×10^6/uL	
Hb	12.4g/dL	10.2g/dL
Hct	36.4%	33.3%
PLT	364%	
BUN	10 mg/dL	
Creatinine	0.5 mg/L	
AST	22 U/L	
Sodium	138 mEq/L	
Potassium	4.0 mEq/L	

Radiology & Image Reports:

1. EGD:
   (1) No visible lesions in esophagus.
   (2) Patchy hyperemia at the body of stomach without any visible lesions.
   (3) No visible lesions in duodenum.
   Diagnosis: Superficial gastritis.
2. CT scan: CT study of the abdomen before and after the use of contrast medium shows:
   (1) No evident dilatation of intrahepatic bile ducts.
   (2) Patent enhancement of the transplanted portal vein.
   (3) No evident abdominal fluid accumulation.
   (4) No evident enlargement of abdominal lymph nodes.

Pathological report:

Nil.

Operation Date, Method and Findings:

Date of operation: 2023/1/13.

Operation performed: Remove a Port-A catheter.

Surgeon: ×××.

Anesthesia: LA-local 0.25% Marcaine.

Estimated blood loss: Minimal.

Blood transfused: None.

Specimens: None.

OP findings: Remove Port-A-Catheter.

Course and treatment:

After admission. This 3 year-old female received operation on 2023/1/13. The patient tolerated the operation smoothly. After the operation, her condition was stable and the wound healed well. Wound pain has relieved after the operation. She now walks smoothly. Thus, with stable condition, she was discharged on 2023/1/14.

Complication:

Nil.

Status on Discharge:

Stable.

Recommendations & Medications:

1. Regular wound care at home and keep dry.
2. OPD follow up 2 weeks later.
3. Cyclosporine A (100 mg/mL) 0.1 mL BID PO.

Attending Physician: ×××

Resident: △△△

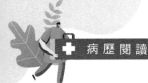

護理小幫手

Little Helper

移植後淋巴異常增生疾病是一種移植後併發症，此病與移植後長期接受免疫抑制治療有關，近年來常使用化學治療合併單株抗體藥物來治療。病童接受治療後出院返家休養，宜注意居家的自我照顧，說明如下：

1. 良好的日常生活照顧：
   (1) 採均衡飲食，少量多餐，且不吃生食。
   (2) 養成良好的衛生習慣、多喝水、常洗手及注意口腔清潔。
   (3) 維持足夠的睡眠及休息。
   (4) 保持皮膚完整性：使用尖銳物品宜小心，避免刺傷、割傷及防碰撞。
   (5) 保持居家環境的通風、乾爽，避免養寵物及室內盆栽。
   (6) 勿接觸感染者，並減少出入公共場所，外出需戴口罩。
2. 放鬆心情，做適當的緩和運動，如聽音樂、散步等。
3. 如有高燒不退、呼吸喘、解血尿、血便、黑便、出血點等狀況，請立即就醫。

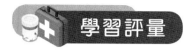 學習評量

一、選擇題

(　)1.　以下何者是病童的主要住院診斷之一？(A)Type 2 DM　(B)Biliary atresia, s/p　(C)URI　(D)Hypoglycemia

(　)2.　請問下列何者不是病童曾做過的手術？(A)Kasai operation　(B)liver transplantation　(C)appendectomy　(D)insert Port-A catheter

(　)3.　病童入院時的血液常規檢查中，有測 EBV viral load，中譯為何？(A)白血球數值　(B)EB 病毒量　(C)血小板數值　(D)感染指數

(　)4.　下列何者為此次病童的入院目的？(A)做切片檢查　(B)行化學治療　(C)B 細胞移植後增生異常復發　(D)移除 Port-A 導管

(　)5.　下列何者為目前病童的主要治療用藥？(A)Cyclosporine A　(B)Ganciclovir　(C)CHOP　(D)抗 CD20 單株抗體

二、配合題

(　)1.　Transplantation
(　)2.　Lymphoproliferative
(　)3.　Jaundice
(　)4.　Biliary atresia
(　)5.　Bilirubin
(　)6.　Chemotherapy
(　)7.　Gastritis
(　)8.　Biopsy
(　)9.　Vaccination
(　)10.　Bone marrow aspiration

(A)化學治療　(J)吞嚥困難
(B)移植　(K)淋巴增生
(C)心臟衰竭　(L)組織切片
(D)骨髓抽吸　(M)三尖瓣
(E)高血鈣　(N)疫苗接種
(F)神經病變　(O)診斷
(G)高血糖　(P)黃疸
(H)胃炎　(Q)低血鈉
(I)膽道閉鎖　(R)膽紅素

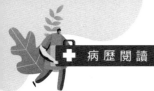
三、填充題

請寫出以下縮寫或生字之全文及中譯。

1. MRCP _____
2. HIDA _____
3. PET _____
4. PTLD _____
5. PROM _____
6. HBV _____
7. WNL _____
8. EGD _____
9. LAP _____
10. RCM _____

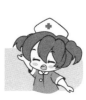

06 | CHAPTER

精神科病歷

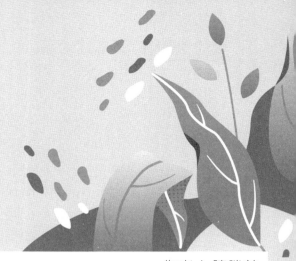

作者｜陳勝美

Admission Note

Progress Note

Order Sheet

Mini-Mental State Examination (MMSE)

Consultation Sheet

Reply Sheet

Discharge Summary

☑ 閱讀導引
1. 了解個案主訴與現在病史的關係。
2. 分析現在病史與過去病史之關聯性。
3. 分析病情與治療措施的合適性。

☑ PREVIEW
閱讀本章前，請讀者先自行預習思覺失調症的相關知識喔！
1. 精神科病歷的記錄重點。
2. 精神狀態的評估與診斷的方式。
3. 思覺失調症之病因、診斷、治療及預後。

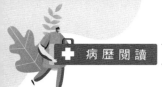

Admission Note

Psychiatric, female, 42 years old, unmarried.

Source of information: The patient and family (middle elder brother).

Date of admission: 2023-1-12.

Identifying Data:

The subject is a 42 year-old high school graduate unmarried female, who was brought to the hospital by one of her elder brothers.

Chief Complaint:

The patient stated: "I hear voices telling me to do bad things. There are often two or three voices talking at the same time, and they often talk to each other." Commenting further on her behavior: "I often hear voices telling me to pinch myself. One time, I got so angry that I threw a house fan because I was tired of hearing the voices. I further think that people are making fun of me when they are not. I also screamed "shut up" at my mom. I cannot go to work because of the voices. I am afraid of these voices". She said she has not been able to sleep well for a long period of time. She has suffered tremendously.

Present Illness:

According to her family, the patient has a long history of schizophrenia which has required hospitalization. However, she had been doing fairly well for the past five years until several months ago, when she lost her work due to the onset, once again, of her illness. This was precipitated by work-related stress. Subsequently, she forgot to take her medication. She avoided contacting with other people, and began "self talking" and making unrealistic plans to become the president of the company. She agreed to this admission on the advice of her elder brother.

Past Psychiatric History:

The patient felt that she had recovered fairly well and believed that this was due to her overall treatment for her schizophrenia. Her condition had markedly improved over the years. According to statements made by her brother, she initially had a fairly good position within SanYang Motor. The company, however, began to reduce its staffing levels; this placed additional pressure on all employees. She could not deal with this and was subsequently terminated. She then got a new position of answering phones. She also failed at this position. Her final job consisted of being an office cleaner. With the onset of her disease (at the age of 37), she also lost this work. After lengthy periods of hospitalization, she was finally deemed healthy enough to continue her treatment as a hospital outpatient. Her diagnosis and treatment included the oral consumption of Risdol (2 mg) 1# QN on a regular basis. Her brother stated that until her last job dismissal, she had regularly visited the outpatient services and had taken her medication, losing her job had, therefore, once again, presented clearly analyzable self-talking symptoms and violent behavior.

Personal History:

The subject is a 42 year-old high school graduate, unmarried female, no smoking, no alcohol drinking, no food allergies, no drug allergies, no substance related disorders.

Social History:

The patient grew up in a farming family and has three older brothers. Her parents are elderly. Thus, her 50 year-old middle older brother is her principal caregiver who stated that "Since her early childhood, she had always been considered to be very clever. She was, however, the only daughter and did not have other local female playmates. This produced severe loneliness and, in her desire for companionship, her initial state of self talking began. This continued in high school and later when she went to work. She had always felt lonely and said that people gossiped behind her back."

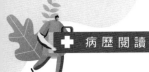

Family History:

Her youngest elder brother has also displayed signs of **psychosis** still hospitalization. No cancer, DM, heart diseases, **hypertension, CVA**, liver diseases, hepatitis B and kidney disease histories were noted among the family members.

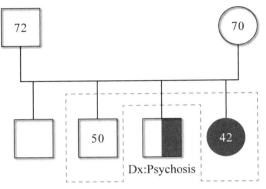

註：個案三哥也患有精神病(psychosis)。

Mental Status Examination:

1. Appearance: Appropriate.
2. Attitude: Distant.
3. Conscious: Clear.
4. **Speech**: Incoherent.
5. Affect & mood: Apathetic.
6. Behavior: Self-talking.
7. Thought: **Delusion of reference**.
8. **Perception**: **AH**

9. **JOMAC**:
   (1) Judgment: Impaired.
   (2) Orientation: Normal.
   (3) Memory: Impaired memory.
   (4) Abstract thinking: Poor.
   (5) Calculation: Impaired.
10. **Insight**: Poor.

病歷小幫手   Little Helper

精神科病歷的記錄書寫

由於精神科病人求診時會受到疾病症狀的干擾而無法正確或完整的表達其主述，可由其家屬或照顧者提供更多訊息。但盡量還是要以病人為主要對象來探討其問題核心。在評估精神疾病的同時也需一併評估其他系統的內外科問題。

醫護人員在記錄時可以同時將病人與家屬或照顧者的主述一併記錄，但須以其主訴為記錄文字，而非以專業名詞來記錄。例如本個案主訴提到「我聽見聲音叫我去做『壞事』。經常有二～三種的聲音同時在談話」。醫師不會書寫成「病人主訴有幻聽干擾」。

關鍵字彙 Keywords

字　彙	原　文	中　譯
Psychosis		精神病
Hypertension	hyper-，過、多、高	高血壓
CVA	cerebrovascular accident	腦血管意外、腦中風
Speech		言語
Delusion of reference	delusion，妄想	關係妄想
Perception		知覺
AH	auditory hallucinations	幻聽
JOMAC	judgement, orientation, memory, abstract thinking, calculation	判斷力、定向感、記憶力、抽象思考、計算力
Insight		病識感

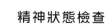

護理小幫手

Little Helper

精神狀態檢查

1. 意識狀態：一般內外科病人在意識方面的評估會著重在神經學方面的評估，但精神科的意識評估尚須包含病人對外在環境的反應，如恐慌症病人意識處於過度警醒狀態的描述。

2. 外表、態度：例如病人看起來敵視、防衛心很重、非常熱絡、友善，外表儀容是否恰當等。

3. 情感和心情：包括是否病人情感表達適切，冷淡或過於熱情，以及情緒是否穩定等。

4. 思考語言：是否有妄想、思考脫軌、思考鬆散、知覺障礙等情形。

5. 行為症狀：例如自言自語、激躁不安、攻擊、自傷或自殺等行為。通常行為症狀會是家屬求助就醫的主要原因。

6. JOMAC。

7. 病識感。

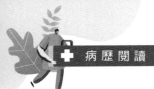

Laboratory:

1. CBC

Date	RBC	WBC	Hb	Hct	MCV	MCHC
2023/1/12	$4.55 \times 10^6/\mu L$	6,000/μL	12.9 g/dL	38.2%	89.3 fL	33.8%

2. Differential Count

Date	Lymphocytes	Monocytes	Eosinophils	Basophils	HBsAg
2023/1/12	37.6%	6.4%	6.6%	3.1%	(+)

3. BCS

Date	T_4
2023/1/12	14.4

Assessment:

The patient exhibits poor sleep patterns, self-talking, delusions of reference, AH (auditory hallucinations) and **loosening of association**. The symptoms have continued for several months.

Diagnosis:

Schizophrenia.

Therapeutic Plan:

1. Psychiatric ward admission routine.
2. Administration of antipsychotic medications to alleviate her psychotic symptoms.
3. Functional rehabilitation program.
4. Family **psychoeducation**.

Attending Physician: ×××

Resident: △△△

護理小幫手

Little Helper

臨床上常用簡易的 JOMAC 來測試及表現病人的智能狀況，包括：

1. 判斷力(Judgement)：正確評估情境並做適當反應的能力，例如「失火時該如何處理」。

2. 定向感(Orientation)：對人、時、地的正確認知程度。

3. 記憶力(Memory)：可以根據記憶事件的遠近分為立即(immediate)、近期(recent)、遠期(remote)等。

4. 抽象思考(Abstract thinking)：運用多方面認知來了解抽象概念及隱喻，並做成適當結論的能力。

5. 計算力(Calculation)：常用問題如「100 減 7 減五次，共有五個答案，請你一個一個回答。」

關鍵字彙 Keywords

字 彙	原 文	中 譯
Loosening of association	Loosening，鬆弛、鬆動 Association，聯想、聯合	聯想鬆弛
Schizophrenia		思覺失調症
Psychoeducation	Psycho-，心理 Education，教育	心理衛生教育

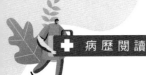

護理小幫手

Little Helper

《精神疾病診斷與統計手冊》(The Diagnostic and Statistical Manual of Mental Disorders, DSM)－是用來診斷精神疾病的指導手冊，由美國精神醫學學會出版。精神疾病診斷統計手冊第五版(DSM-5)為目前美國精神醫學會及國內多數臨床精神科所使用之診斷準則，DSM-5 考慮到因為牽涉保險給付、擔心獨立出第二軸易造成疾病汙名化等原因，目前已經取消五軸診斷。

ICD 疾病分類系統(International Statistical Classification of Diseases and Related Health Problems, ICD)是由聯合國世界衛生組織(WHO)出版的「國際疾病分類系統」。ICD 系統涵蓋身體所有系統的疾病，精神疾病只是其中的一部分，在台灣健保醫療系統因方便申請健保給付，故臨床上皆以 ICD 進行診斷，而非 DSM。

Progress Note

Psychiatric, female, 42 years old, unmarried.

Source of information: The patient and family.

Date of admission: 2023-1-12.

2023-1-12

#1 Due to auditory hallucinations change patient's emotional state and behavior

S:

1. Poor sleep.
2. Hearing two or more voices conversing with each other.
3. The voices telling me to do "bad things".
4. Tired and be scared of those voices.
5. They said "I am a bad girl" made me angry and fear.

O:

1. Vital signs: BT: 36.2°C, PR: 64/min, RR: 24/min, BP: 126/78 mmHg.
2. Frequently self-talking.
3. Total sleep time: 4~5 hrs/day.
4. Affect: **Anxiety.**
5. Behavior: **Withdraw.**
6. Poor attention: Only a few second or minutes.

A: Due to auditory hallucinations change patient's emotional state and behavior.

P:

1. Risdol (2 mg) 1# **HS** PO.
2. Limin (5 mg) 1# **QN** PO.
3. Gradually titrate Risdol: Monitor closely and observe the efficacy.

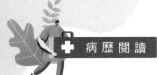

4. Accept client as they are and encourages expression of feelings.

5. Psycho education: Improve insight.

6. Interview and evaluation hallucinations themselves.

2023/1/13

#2 Increase autonomic nervous system signs of anxiety, such as heart rate, respiration, blood pressure and difficulty relating to others

S:

1. **Insomnia.**

2. Feeling loss of control.

3. Filled with guilt.

O:

1. Vital signs: BT: 37.2°C, PR: 94/min, RR: 28/min, BP: 136/80 mmHg.

2. Serious anxiety.

3. Difficulty relating to others.

4. Behavior: Violence.

A: Increased autonomic nervous system signs of anxiety, such as heart rate, respiration, blood pressure and difficulty relating to others.

P: Titrate: Risdol to 4 mg once a day, add Bipiden 2 mg once a day.

1. Risdol (2 mg) 1# BID PO.

2. Bipiden (2 mg) 1# QD PO.

2023/1/14

＃3 No reality, no safety, and maladaptive

S:

1. Poor sleep.
2. Loneliness.
3. Can not manage anxiety.

O:

1. Vital signs: BT: 36.2°C, PR: 74/min, RR: 20/min, BP: 126/80 mmHg.
2. No **EPS**.
3. Thought: loosing of association.
4. Insight: Impaired.
5. Self-talking, but no violence.
6. Restricted affect.

A: No reality, no safety, and maladaptive.

P:

1. Risdol (2 mg) 1# QD PO.
2. Risdol (2 mg) 2# HS PO.
3. B.H.L (5 mg) 1# QD PO.
4. Supportive **psychotherapy**.
5. Improve reality.
6. Improve insight.

Attending Physician: ×××

Resident: △△△

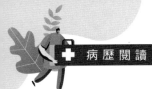

病歷閱讀 | Understanding Medical Records

關鍵字彙 Keywords

字　彙	原　文	中　譯
Anxiety		焦慮
Withdraw		退縮
HS	L. *hora somni*, at bed time	睡前
QN	L. *quaque nocte*, every night	每晚
Insomnia		失眠
EPS	extrapyramidal syndrome	錐體外徑症候群
Psychotherapy	psycho-，心理 -therapy，治療	心理治療

 Thinking About

1. 為何醫師需要不斷調整個案的用藥？
2. 除了藥物治療之外，精神科復健的部分醫師做了哪些安排？

Order Sheet

Psychiatric, female, 42 years old, unmarried.

Source of information: The patient and family.

Date of admission: 2023-1-12.

Standing Order

2023-1-12

Diagnosis: Schizophrenia and DM

1. On psychiatric ward routine.

2. On regular vital signs.

3. On regular diet.

4. Psychopharmacological treatment: Seven times a week.

5. Specially group psychotherapy: Once a week.

6. Active treatment: Five times a week.

7. Psychiatric general occupational therapy: Eight times a week.

8. Family therapy: Twice a month.

9. Supporting psychotherapy: Twice a week.

10. Assessment of social life function: Once a month.

11. Check physiological and psychological function: Twice a month.

Medications:

1. Risdol (2 mg) 1# HS PO.

2. Limin (5 mg) 1# QN PO.

2023/1/13

1. Risdol (2 mg) 1# BID PO.

2. Bipiden (2 mg) 1# QD PO.

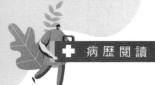

2023/1/14

1. Risdol (2 mg) 1# QD PO.

2. Risdol (2 mg) 2# HS PO.

3. B.H.L. (5 mg) 1# QD PO.

4. MgO 1# TID PO.

Attending Physician: ×××

Resident: △△△

Stat Order

2023/1/12

1. Check CBC+DC ×1 stat.

2. Biochemistry Examination: AC, BUN, Creatinine, AST, ALT, Na, K, Cl, T_4, Albumin, Bilirubin T/D, TC, TG.

3. Serum test: VDRL、HBsAg、Amebic antigen test.

4. Urine routine examination.

5. EKG.

6. Chest X-ray (PA).

2023/1/14

1. Consulting psychologist.

2023/1/15

1. Consulting occupational therapist.

2023/1/16

1. Consulting social worker.

Attending Physician: ×××

Resident: △△△

Mini-Mental State Examination (MMSE)

項目	分數	測驗得分	測驗內容
A.定向感	5	4	現在時間：<u>冬季</u>、民國 <u>112</u> 年、<u>1</u> 月、<u>10</u> 日、星期<u>?</u>
	5	3	現在居住地方：<u>台中市</u>、<u>北區</u>、<u>文心路</u>、<u>?</u>號、<u>?</u>樓
B.注意力	3	3	請注意聽我說三個詞，結束時請複述一次： 個案回答三個詞是：<u>腳踏車</u>、<u>快樂</u>、<u>紅色</u>
C.計算力	5	3	100 減 7 = <u>93</u>；93 減 7 = <u>86</u>；86 減 7 = <u>79</u>； 再減=<u>?</u>、<u>?</u>、<u>?</u>
D.記憶	3	1	您記得剛剛在計算數字之前說的三個詞嗎？ 個案回答：<u>剛才的三種腳踏車</u>、<u>?</u>、<u>?</u>
E.語言	2	2	分別指著手錶、鉛筆問這是什麼： 個案回答：<u>手錶</u>、<u>鉛筆</u>
	1	1	請重複等一下我說的話：「沒來有往不自在。」 個案復述：<u>沒來有往不自在</u>
	3	3	請說和做以下的動作「閉上眼睛」 個案唸出並照做
	1	1	請寫句子（含文意，多於 3 個字）： 個案寫出：<u>今天要看醫生</u>
	1	1	照我說的做三個動作： 個案照做：<u>手拿紙</u>、<u>折成一半</u>、<u>交給我</u>
	1	1	畫圖：請抄繪圖圖形 個案畫的圖：　⬭⬭

檢查結果：得分 23/30，個案認知功能為輕度失智。

施測者：○○○

評分方面滿分是 30 分。國際標準 24 分為分界值，18~24 分為輕度失智，16~17 分為中度失智，≦15 分為重度失智。我國因教育程度不同分界值也不同；文盲為 17 分，小學（教育年限≦6 年）為 20 分，中學及以上為 24 分。

資料來源：

1. 郭乃文、劉秀枝、王珮芳、徐道昌(1989)．簡短式智能評估(MMSE)之簡介．*臨床醫學月刊*，*23*(1)，39-42。

2. Folstein, M., Folstein, S., McHugh, P. (1975) . "Mini-mental state": A practical method for grading the cognitive state of patients for the clinician. *J Psychiat Res*, *12*, 189-198.

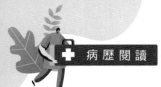

Consultation Sheet

姓名：○○○　　　性別：女　　　出生日期：****-*-*　　病歷號碼：××××××

入院日期：2023-1-12　床號：××　　開單科別：精神科　　照會科別：整形外科

This is a 42 year-old female, who is a schizophrenia patient with DM. She injured her right hand by herself about one week ago and the wound was sutured at that time. Now the wound condition is poor. We need your help for further evaluation.

Dr. ××× at 2023-1-12 1:00 p.m.

- -

Reply Sheet

Dear Dr. ×××,

Local cellulitis & skin defect s/p suture over right hand along 5th metacarpal area 5×5 cm. Suggestion :

1. Soaking with Normal saline BID.

2. Control DM.

3. Elevation of R't hand with pillow.

4. X-ray if R't hand R/O fracture.

5. Oral or IV antibiotics.

Dr. ○○○ at 2023-1-12 3:00 p.m.

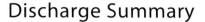

Discharge Summary

Psychiatric, female, 42 years old, unmarried.

Source of information: The patient and family (middle elder brother).

Date of admission: 2023-1-12.

Date of discharge: 2023-1-25.

Admission Diagnosis:

Schizophrenia.

Discharge Diagnosis:

Schizophrenia.

Identifying Data:

The subject is a 42 year-old high school graduate, unmarried female, who was brought to the hospital by one of her elder brothers.

Chief Complaint:

The patient stated: "I hear voices telling me to do bad things. There are often two or three voices talking at the same time, and they often talk to each other." Commenting further on her behavior: "I often hear voices telling me to pinch myself. One time, I got so angry that I threw a house fan because I was tired of hearing the voices. I further think that people are making fun of me when they are not. I also screamed "shut up" at my mom. I cannot go to work because of the voices. I am afraid of these voices". She said she has not been able to sleep well for a long period of time. She has suffered tremendously.

Brief History:

According to her family, the patient has a long history of schizophrenia which has required hospitalization. However, she had been doing fairly well for the past five years until several months ago, when she lost her work due to the onset, once again, of her illness. This was

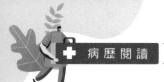

precipitated by work-related stress. Subsequently, she forgot to take her medication. She avoided contacting with other people, and began "self talking" and making unrealistic plans to become the president of the company. She agreed to this admission on the advice of her elder brother.

Physical Findings:

Nil.

Course and Treatment:

The patient responded well to individual and group psychotherapy, milieu therapy and medication management. As stated, family therapy was conducted.

1. Psychopharmacologic management.
2. Individual and group psychotherapy.
3. Family therapy conducted by social work department, with the patient and the patient's family, for the purpose of education and discharge planning.

Laboratory:

1. CBC

Date	RBC	WBC	Hb	Hct	MCV	MCHC
2023/1/12	$4.55 \times 10^6/\mu L$	6,000/μL	12.9 g/dL	38.2%	89.3 fL	33.8%

2. Differential count

Date	Lymphocytes	Monocytes	Eosinophils	Basophils	HBsAg
2023/1/12	37.6%	6.4%	6.6%	3.1%	(+)

3. BCS

Date	T_4
2023/1/12	14.4

Complications:

Nil.

Status on Discharge:

Stable. Discharge instructions/routine for medical outpatient services.

Discharge Order:

1. Risdol (2 mg) 1# HS PO.
2. B.H.L. (5 mg) 1# QD PO.
3. MgO 1# TID PO.
4. To return in one month for OPD follow up.

Attending Physician: ×××

Resident: △△△

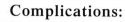

護理小幫手

Little Helper

　　協助思覺失調症病人與家屬面對疾病及生活適應，是精神醫療服務重要的一環。護理人員可教導病人情緒與疾病上的管理、加強人際互動技巧訓練，並依個別需求，給予相關的護理措施，包括：

1. 加強病識感，建立規則服藥的習慣，並告知「不可自行停藥或減藥」的重要性。
2. 安排規律生活作息，學習壓力因應技巧，如放鬆技巧、聽音樂等緩解壓力。
3. 定期返診，適時與醫師討論病情、用藥劑量、服藥次數等。
4. 若發覺睡眠情況變差、精神症狀加劇，服藥遵從性差且影響生活品質，應盡快返診求治，預防再度復發。
5. 鼓勵家屬參加支持性團體，分享彼此的經驗，學習專業知識，相互提供情緒支持，同時也提升病人及家屬的照護品質。

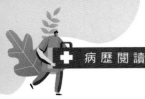

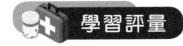

一、選擇題

(　　)1.　以下何者不是個案出現的症狀？(A)Self talking　(B)Loosening of association (C)Auditory hallucination　(D)Hypoglycemia

(　　)2.　請問個案的 Mental Status Examination 評估中，下列何者為非？(A)Speech: Incoherent　(B)Judgment: Normal　(C)Memory: Impaired memory (D)Insight: Poor

(　　)3.　下列與個案有關的敘述何者為非？(A)Her youngest elder brother has also displayed signs of psychosis.　(B)She was, however, the only daughter and did not have other local female playmates.　(C)Patient has a long history of schizophrenia and never get treatment.　(D)The patient hear voices telling her to do bad things.

(　　)4.　下列何者是個案的臨床精神疾病診斷？(A)Schizophrenia　(B)DM (C)Personality Disorder　(D)Depression

(　　)5.　請問此個案的 MMSE 評估結果為何？(A)認知功能受損　(B)輕度認知功能 受損　(C)認知功能正常　(D)無法評估

二、配合題

( )1. Schizophrenia

( )2. Substance related disorders

( )3. Speech

( )4. Judgment

( )5. Orientation

( )6. Anxiety

( )7. Loosening of association

( )8. DSM-5

( )9. Conscious

( )10. Auditory hallucinations

(A)簡短智能測驗

(B)思覺失調症

(C)錯覺

(D)精神疾病診斷與統計手冊第五版

(E)認知障礙

(F)意識

(G)高血糖

(H)物質相關障礙症

(I)言語

(J)憂鬱症

(K)判斷力

(L)幻聽

(M)定向感

(N)手術

(O)焦慮

(P)低血糖

(Q)聯想鬆弛

(R)說話困難

學習評量解答
請掃描 QR Code

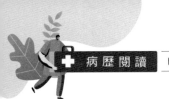
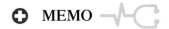
MEMO

07 | CHAPTER

急症病歷

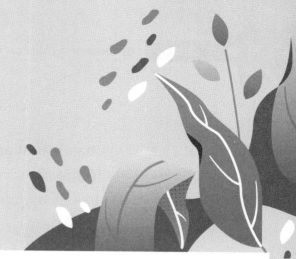

作者｜薛承君、劉明德
Jonathan Seak

ED Chart
Order Sheet
Laboratory Results
Imaging Report
Observation Order
Sputum Culture
ED Progress Note
Order Sheet
Central Line Insertion Procedure Note
Imaging Report
ED Consultation Sheet
Consultation Reply Sheet

☑ 閱讀導引

1. 了解急診病歷之特色及閱讀時該注意的事項。
2. 了解閱讀及執行急診醫囑時該注意的事項。
3. 了解個案的病史與發病過程。
4. 了解個案病程發展及相關治療的關聯。
5. 能判讀個案各種檢驗及檢查結果的意義。
6. 能掌握閱讀會診單及照會回覆單之重點。

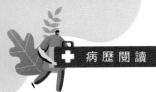

ED Chart

Name: ○○○　　　Chart Number: ×××××　　Sex: Male　　Age : 57

Bed No: ××　　　**Triage**: ××　　Time of Arrival: 2023/3/26 17:00

Method of Arrival: Sent by family

BT: 39.2°C　　HR: 100/min　　RR: 20/min

BP: 108/88 mmHg　　**GCS**: $E_4V_5M_6$　　SpO$_2$: 92%

Chief Complaint:

Fever for 1 day.

Present Illness:

A 57 year-old man was brought in by his son. Cough and **runny nose** for 1 week.

Yellowish sputum was noted for 2 days.

Fever started since the night before.

Associated with shortness of breath.

No **orthopnea**, no **PND**, no **palpitation**. No sorethroat, no headache, no ear pain.

No **dysuria**, no urinary frequency, no urinary urgency, no **flank pain**.

No abdominal pain, no nausea, no vomiting, no constipation, no diarrhea.

Past Medical and Personal History:

1. **Diabetes mellitus** for 10 years under regular **OHA** control.
2. Denied recent history of travelling.

Medication History:

1. Glipizide 1# QD PO.
2. Metformin 1# TID PO.
3. No known allergies.

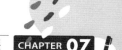

 ## 關鍵字彙 Keywords

字　彙	原　文	中　譯
Triage		檢傷分類級數
GCS	Glasgow coma scale	格拉斯哥昏迷指數
Runny nose		流鼻水
Orthopnea		端坐呼吸
PND	paroxysmal nocturnal dyspnea	陣發性夜間呼吸困難
Palpitation		心悸
Dysuria		少尿
Flank pain		腰痛
Diabetes mellitus (DM)		糖尿病
OHA	oral hypoglycemic agents	口服降血糖藥物

 ## 病歷小幫手

Little Helper

　　以上是病人抵院時急診病歷之一般書寫方式。病歷之第一行記載了病人之姓名、病歷號碼、性別、年齡等基本資料，以供急診醫護人員辨識；由於每種疾病之盛行率在不同性別之年齡層大有不同，這些基本資料可供醫護人員做初步鑑別診斷之依據。

　　病歷第二行記載了病人在急診的病床位置、檢傷分類級數(triage)及到院時間。目前國內急診之檢傷系統是採用五級檢傷分類，依病人到院時急診病情之嚴重度分為五級；最嚴重（如心跳停止、呼吸衰竭）為第一級病人，最輕症（如鼻胃管滑脫，要求重新放置）為第五級；我們這位病人之檢傷分類級數為第三級，意即中度嚴重病人。急診室病人的處置原則是嚴重度越高之病人優先診治，所以病歷上之檢傷分類級數就提供了急診醫護人員在選擇處置病人順序上良好的資訊。

　　接下來的病歷第四至五行，是病人到院時之生命徵象，包括體溫、脈搏、呼吸、血壓、意識狀態、周邊血氧濃度等數據，可以判定病人是否需先施予急救或緊急處理。

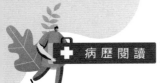

Physical Examination:

1. BT: 39.2°C, HR: 100 beats/min, RR: 20 breaths/min, BP: 108/88 mmHg, SpO_2: 92%.

2. General appearance: Acutely ill-looking. Consciousness: Alert and responsive.

3. HEENT: Pupils: +3/+3, pink conjunctiva. Sclera: anicteric, throat: Not erythematous.

4. Neck: Supple, no **lymphadenopathy**, no **JVE**.

5. Chest: Symmetrical expansion, **bilateral basal crackles**, mild wheezing.

6. Heart: Regular rate and rhythm, no murmur.

7. Abdomen: Soft and flat, normoactive bowel sounds, no tenderness, no **hepatospleno-megaly**.

8. Back: No **costovertebral angle** knocking pain.

9. Extremities: Freely movable, no leg **pitting edema**.

10. Skin: No lesion.

Impression:

1. **Pneumonia**.
2. Diabetes mellitus.

Management:

1. O_2 cannula 5 L/min.
2. Check CBC/DC, finger stick blood sugar, AST/ALT, BUN/Cr., Na/K.
3. **Arterial blood gas** analysis.
4. Blood cultures×2.
5. IVF with N/S run 60 mL/hr.
6. Sputum smear and culture.
7. Chest X-ray.
8. Empirical antibiotics.

Attending Physician: ○○○

2023/3/26　17:28

關鍵字彙 Keywords

字　彙	原　文	中　譯
Lymphadenopathy	lymph-，淋巴 -adeno，腺 -pathy，病變	淋巴腺病變、淋巴腺腫大
JVE	jugular vein engorgement	頸靜脈怒張
Bilateral basal crackles		雙側肺底部有爆裂音
Hepatosplenomegaly		肝脾腫大
Costovertebral angle		肋脊角
Pitting edema		凹陷性水腫
Pneumonia	pneumo-，肺	肺炎
Arterial blood gas (ABG)		動脈血液氣體

病歷小幫手

Little Helper

　　緊接之病歷寫作內容是依照主訴→現在病史→過去醫療史及個人史→藥物史→身體檢查→臆斷→處置等大方向進行記錄。病人之主訴相當清楚，即發燒一天；這簡明扼要說明了病人求診原因。接下來的病史部分是以條列方式書寫，記載了病症開始之時間（咳嗽一星期），為何會被帶至急診（昨夜開始發燒，併有呼吸困難之情形），病人同時合併之其他症狀（有黃痰）。而在過去醫療史及個人史之部分，則是條列式地載明了病人之糖尿病已有 10 年歷史；藥物史方面，則扼要記載使用 Glipizide 及 Metformin 等兩種口服降血糖藥之方式，同時說明病人沒有藥物或食物過敏史。

　　在身體檢查方面，清楚記載了與主訴有關之特別發現：包括發燒（體溫 39.2℃）、心跳快（每分鐘 100 下）、呼吸急促（每分鐘 20 下）、周邊血氧濃度較低(92%)、病人有急性病態外觀、雙側肺底部有爆裂音及喘鳴聲等。最後才依病人問題之嚴重緊迫性依序作出(1)肺炎、(2)糖尿病等診斷臆測。另外針對病情，也做出相對應之處置包括給予氧氣、抽血檢驗、送痰液及血液細菌培養、照胸部 X 光及給予抗生素等措施。最後，負責診治之醫師在病歷記載後也進行了簽章併註明記載時間，如此急診病歷方告一段落。

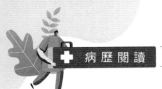

Order Sheet

Name: ○○○　　　Chart Number: ×××××　　　Sex: Male　　Age: 57

Bed No: ××

1. O_2 cannula 5 L/ min.
2. CBC.
3. WBC differential count.
4. Finger stick sugar stat.
5. AST (GOT).
6. ALT (GPT).
7. Blood urea nitrogen (BUN).
8. Cr. (Creatinine).
9. Na (Sodium).
10. K (Potassium).
11. Arterial blood gas analysis.
12. **Common aerobic culture** (SP).
13. **Gram stain** (SP).
14. **Acid fast stain** (SP).
15. **Blood culture** (1st).
16. Blood culture (2nd).
17. Chest X-ray A-P view (Supine).
18. **Penicillin Skin Test** stat.
19. IVF with N/S mL run 60 mL/hr.
20. Augmentin Inj (Amoxicillin 500 mg + Clavulanic Acid 100 mg) 1.2 g IVF stat.

Attending Physician: ○○○

2023/3/26 17:38:25

關鍵字彙 Keywords

字　彙	中　譯
Common aerobic culture	一般嗜氧培養
Gram stain	革蘭氏染色
Acid fast stain	抗酸性染色
Blood culture	血液培養
Penicillin Skin Test (PST)	盤尼西林皮膚測試

護理小幫手

Little Helper

　　上述醫囑是針對病人來急診時所做之處置，由於病人主訴發燒，有咳嗽併黃痰且有呼吸困難之情形，在身體檢查方面有高燒（體溫 39.2℃）、心搏加速（100 次／分鐘）、偏喘（20 次／分鐘）、周邊血氧濃度降低（SpO$_2$：92%）之情形，且肺部之雙側底部有爆裂音及喘鳴聲，臨床上之診斷臆測主要優先考慮肺炎之可能性，所以處置上亦應依此方向做抽血檢驗（包括全血、生化檢測），血液、痰液細菌培養及胸部 X 光檢查、加以確診及治療，如此才能依 SOAP 之思維解決病人之臨床問題。

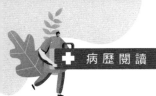
Laboratory Results

姓名：○○○　　　病歷號碼：××××××　　性別：男　　　　　年齡：57
急診床號：××　　　檢體別：血液　　　採檢日期／時間：2023/03/26 17:50
醫囑醫師：○○○　　　　　　　　　　　送檢日期／時間：2023/03/26 18:00
　　　　　　　　　　　　　　　　　　　報告日期／時間：2023/03/26 19:08

Item	Data		Reference Range
WBC	15.6	10^3/uL	M　3.9~10.6
			F　3.5~11
RBC	3.81	10^6/uL	M　4.3~6.1
			F　3.9~5.4
Hemoglobin	12.1	g/dL	M　13.5~17.5
			F　12~16
Hematocrit	35.4	%	M　41~53
			F　36~46
MCV	92.9	fL	80~100
MCH	31.8	pg/Cell	26~34
MCHC	34.2	gHb/dL	31~37
RDW-SD	48.2	fL	38~47.5
Platelets	393	10^3/uL	150~400
RDW-CV	14.2	%	11.0~14.7
Segment	93.1	%	42~74
Lymphocyte	3.3	%	20~56
Monocyte	3.6	%	0~12
Eosinophil	0.0	%	0~5
Basophil	0.0	%	0~1
AST/GOT	27	U/L	0~37
ALT/GPT	38	U/L	0~40
BUN(B)	20	mg/dL	7~20

Item	Data		Reference Range
Creatinine(B)	0.76	mg/dL	M　0.64~1.27
			F　　0.44~1.03
Sodium	135	mEq/L	134~148
Potassium	4.6	mEq/L	3.6~5.0

護理小幫手

Little Helper

　　以上是病人之檢驗報告，在此報告中可見白血球(WBC) 15,600/mm^3，高於參考值之數據，且節狀核嗜中性球較多(Seg: 93%)，這代表病人身體極有可能正受細菌感染或處在生理壓力之下。其餘抽血檢驗報告包括肝功能(AST/ALT)、腎功能(BUN/Cr.)指數、血鈉(Na)、血鉀(K)皆正常，此檢驗數值代表病人雖然身處肺炎感染，但未嚴重至肝腎衰竭或電解質失調。

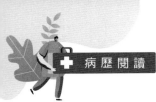
Imaging Report

2023/3/26 CXR

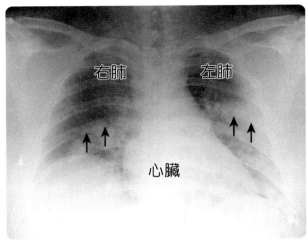

右肺　　左肺

心臟

圖 7-1　病人抵達急診時之胸部 X 光

護理小幫手

Little Helper

　　這是病人到急診時之胸部 X 光，箭頭所指之白色浸潤處為異常之處，在本個案中最有可能之影像異常成因為肺炎，這也和一開始急診醫師之診斷臆測相符。

Observation Order

Name: ○○○　　　Chart Number: ×××××　　Sex: Male　　Age : 57

Bed No: ED OBS ××

Admit to Chest ward under Dr. ○○○.

Diagnosis:　(1) Bilateral Pneumonia.

　　　　　　(2) Diabetes Mellitus.

Vital sign: Q8H.

O$_2$ cannula 5 L/min.

Diet as tolerated.

IVF with N/S run 60 mL/hr.

Medications:

1. Augmentin Inj (Amoxicillin 500 mg + Clavulanic Acid 100 mg) 1.2 g Q8H IVF.
2. Acetaminophen (500) mg/Tab 1# QID PO.
3. Brown Mixture liquid 10 mL QID PO.

Attending Physician: ○○○

2023/3/26 19:48:33

護理小幫手

Little Helper

由於臨床上病人之病史、身體檢查、檢驗及檢查報告皆指向其受肺炎侵襲，故住院治療是必要的；然而，有時住院病房之床位並非馬上即可轉入，這時往往就需先至急診觀察室等侯住院併加以治療，此時就會開立類似上列之急診觀察室醫囑，將病人由急診現場轉至急診觀察室繼續治療。

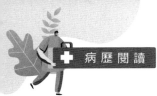

Sputum Culture

姓名：○○○　　　病歷號碼：×××××　　　性別／出生日期：M/****/**/**(57)

病人來源：急診　　病床號：××　　　　　採檢日期／時間：2023/03/26/18:08

醫囑醫師：○○○　　科別：急診內科　　　送檢日期／時間：2023/03/26/18:28

檢驗組別：微生物　　檢體別：SP　　　　報告日期／時間：2023/03/27/06:52

檢體別說明：痰液　　　　　　　　　　　醫囑日期／時間：2023/03/26/17:38

細菌名稱	生長狀態	
1. *Kleb. pneumoniae*	Moderate	
藥敏試驗	1（濃度）	
Ampicillin	.	
Amikacin	. S	
Ceftazidime	. S	
Clindamycin	.	
Ciprofloxacin	. S	
Ceftriaxone	. S	
Cefuroxime	. S	
Cefazolin	. S	
Erythromycin	.	
Ertapenem	. S	
Gentamicin	. S	
Levofloxacin	. S	
Penicillin	.	
Ampicillin-sulbactam	. S	
Sulfamethoxazole-Trimethoprim	. S	
Teicoplanin		
Piperacillin-tazobactam	. S	
Vancomycin	.	

註：S: Sensitive，代表該藥對所培養之細菌有效。

護理小幫手

Little Helper

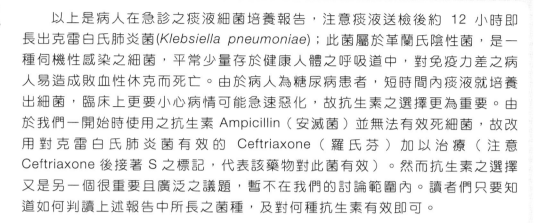

　　以上是病人在急診之痰液細菌培養報告，注意痰液送檢後約 12 小時即長出克雷白氏肺炎菌(*Klebsiella pneumoniae*)；此菌屬於革蘭氏陰性菌，是一種伺機性感染之細菌，平常少量存於健康人體之呼吸道中，對免疫力差之病人易造成敗血性休克而死亡。由於病人為糖尿病患者，短時間內痰液就培養出細菌，臨床上更要小心病情可能急速惡化，故抗生素之選擇更為重要。由於我們一開始時使用之抗生素 Ampicillin（安滅菌）並無法有效死細菌，故改用對克雷白氏肺炎菌有效的 Ceftriaxone（羅氏芬）加以治療（注意 Ceftriaxone 後接著 S 之標記，代表該藥物對此菌有效）。然而抗生素之選擇又是另一個很重要且廣泛之議題，暫不在我們的討論範圍內。讀者們只要知道如何判讀上述報告中所長之菌種，及對何種抗生素有效即可。

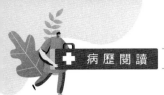

ED Progress Note

Name: ○○○　　　Chart Number: ×××××　　　Sex: Male　　　Age : 57

Bed No: ED OBS ××

#1 Pneumonia (*K.P*) with <u>septic shock</u>

S: Feeling worse this morning. Increase cough with sputum.

O:

1. BT: 38.5°C, HR: 118 beats/min, RR: 22 breaths/min, BP: 86/55 mmHg, SpO_2: 92%.

2. Acutely ill-looking. Consciousness: Alert and orientated.

3. Chest: Crackles over bilateral lower lungs, increased in intensity compared to yesterday.

4. Sputum culture (2023/3/27): *K.P*, sensitive to Ceftriaxone.

A: Pneumonia (*K. P*) with septic shock.

P:

1. Change the antibiotic to Ceftriaxone.

2. <u>Fluid resuscitation</u>. Put on <u>central line</u> for fluid status monitoring.

3. Follow-up chest X-ray.

4. <u>On critical</u> condition. Explain the possibility of <u>respiratory failure</u> to the family.

- -

#2 Diabetes mellitus

S: None.

O: Finger stick blood sugar a.c. / p.c. → 122/168 mg/dL.

A: The <u>hyperglycemia</u> on the day of admission may be due to pneumonia.

P: Keep the present OHA (Glipizide 1 PC QD and Metformin 1 PC TID).

Attending Physician: ○○○

2023/3/27 07:00

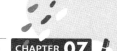

 關鍵字彙 Keywords

字　彙	原　文	中　譯
Septic shock		敗血性休克
K. P	*Klebsiella pneumoniae*	克雷白氏肺炎菌
Fluid resuscitation		灌液復甦
central line		中心靜脈導管
On critical		通知病危
Respiratory failure		呼吸衰竭
Hyperglycemia	hyper-，高 -glyc，糖 -emia，血	高血糖

病歷小幫手

Little Helper

　　以上之急診病程記錄仍然是依照病人問題嚴重性之優先順序加以記載，在此個案中，肺炎之變化就較糖尿病之問題相對來得重要，故優先予以記錄。請注意肺炎及糖尿病這兩個問題之記錄還是以問題導向方式(SOAP)之方式加以書寫，在第一個肺炎之問題中病歷記載了重要之病程身體檢查變化；包括病人之血壓更不穩定(86/55 mmHg)、周邊血氧濃度仍然偏低(92%)、更嚴重的雙肺底部爆裂音等。這些重要發現都要仔細閱讀以掌握病情。除此之外，我們也要注意特殊之檢驗報告結果（痰液培養：克雷白氏肺炎菌）及特殊處置（將抗生素改成 Ceftriaxone、灌液復甦、注射中心靜脈以監測體液之狀況、追蹤 X 光片）和病人動向之改變（發病危通知單，告知家屬會惡化成呼吸衰竭之可能性），以對病情做全盤之了解。

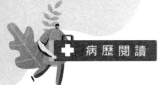
Order Sheet

Name: ○○○　　　Chart Number: ××××××　　　Sex: Male　　　Age : 57

Bed No: ED OBS ××

1. Ceftriaxone 500 mg/vial 2 PC stat.

2. Ceftriaxone 500 mg/vial 2 PC Q12H.

3. IVF challenge with N/S 500 mL stat.

4. IVF with N/S run 120 mL/hr.

5. Recheck BP after IVF challenge with N/S 500 mL stat.

6. Put on right neck **CVP** line.

7. Check CVP stat and Q8H.

8. Wound **CD**, small (<10cm) care with AQ-BI Q3D and PRN.

9. Chest X-ray A-P view (supine) post CVP (portable).

10. On critical condition.

11. BP and **EKG** monitoring.

12. Consult chest physician for chest **ICU**.

Attending Physician: ○○○

2023/3/27 07:13:28

關鍵字彙 Keywords

字　彙	原　文	中　譯
CVP	central venous pressure	CVP 原指中心靜脈壓，但在台灣常被誤用指稱為 CVC（central venous catheter，又稱中心靜脈導管）。其原因為 CVC 屬於血管內管的一種，放置於大靜脈中可以快速注射藥物、輸液或用來測量 CVP，並且兩者發音相去不遠。故在台灣若醫生說「我要幫這位病人放置 CVP」，其實就是要放 CVC（中心靜脈導管）的意思
CD	change dressing	換藥
EKG	electrocardiogram	心電圖
ICU	intensive care unit	加護病房

護理小幫手

Little Helper

　　以上醫囑是針對病人被轉入急診觀察室後病情變化所做之調整，由於病人主觀上覺得咳嗽更厲害，客觀上生命徵象更不穩定（心跳加速，每分鐘 118 下、呼吸急促、血壓下降至 86/55 mmHg），雙肺之爆裂音較之前更為嚴重，且痰液培養亦長出克雷白氏肺炎菌，故可研判病人可能已有肺炎併發敗血性休克之情形，所以此時應該更積極予以液體復甦以維持足夠之組織灌流，避免休克惡化。

　　根據痰液之細菌培養報告結果，我們可精確地針對克雷白氏肺炎菌用藥，故將抗生素改成第三代廣效性頭孢菌素－Ceftriaxone（羅氏芬）。另外，我們插入中心靜脈導管，以利病人之體液監控（如是否處於脫水狀態）。之後，要記得照胸部 X 光以確認靜脈導管位置，避免氣胸等併發症，同時可評估肺炎惡化之程度。

　　除此之外，我們亦必須再將整個病況向家屬解釋清楚，告知病況危急之情形及有可能進展到呼吸衰竭，以讓家屬了解病情，避免不良溝通所產生之醫療糾紛。

　　最後，由於病人病況極度不穩定，已無法在一般病房照顧治療，所以我們照會胸腔內科醫師安排加護病房以利病人進一步之處置。同時，由於病況危急，病人極需要嚴密之機器監控（血壓及心電圖監視器），以備隨時急救。

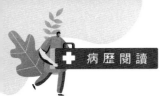

Central Line Insertion Procedure Note

Name: ○○○　　　Chart Number: ✕✕✕✕✕　Sex: Male　　　Age : 57

Bed No: ED OBS ✕✕

Due to septic shock, we inserted a central line for monitoring his fluid status. The patient was lying in a supine position. After local anesthesia, central line was inserted smoothly via the right internal jugular vein. It was fixed at 15 cm. The patient was able to tolerate the procedure well without any complication. Follow-up CXR showed that the central line was in an acceptable position.

Resident Physician: ○○○

2023/3/27 08:00:48

護理小幫手　　　　　　　　　　　　　　　　　　　Little Helper

　　以上是注射中心靜脈導管之過程記錄。一般而言，進行侵入性治療之前，一定要向家屬解釋清楚檢查目的、過程及可能發生之併發症和如何善後，取得同意書後方可進行。然而在非常危急且一時聯絡不上家屬之情況下，可請第三人做見證並簽署醫急醫療見證同意書（在台灣一般是醫院警衛代為見證），以利生命危急之病人的緊急處置。

Imaging Report

2023/3/27 CXR

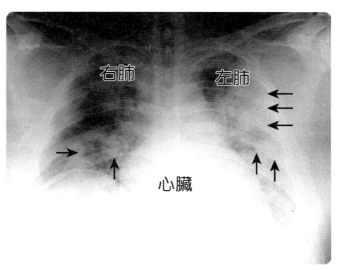

圖 7-2　病人在觀察室時胸部 X 光之追蹤結果

護理小幫手

Little Helper

　　這是病人胸部 X 光之追蹤結果，請注意黑色箭頭所示為肺炎，與入急診時所照之胸部 X 光比較，面積有明顯擴大之情形，這表示病人之病情正逐漸惡化，必須接受更積極之治療及處置。

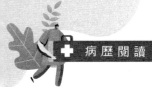
ED Consultation Sheet

姓名：○○○　　病歷號碼：×××××　性別：男　　　　　年齡：57

請求胸腔內科林醫師會診　　日期：2023/3/27 08:30　　☐選擇性 ☑緊急

Present Illness: This is a 57 year-old patient with bilateral pneumonia complicated with septic shock. Please arrange admission to chest ICU for him. Thank you.

Kindly request your
☐Recommendation
☐Diagnosis
☑Treatment
☑Transfer, PRN
☑Discussion
☐Others
Referred from ED.

Resident Physician: ○○○
Attending Physician: × × ×

護理小幫手　Little Helper

　　以上是急診之會診單，與他科醫師合作共同照護病人是急診特色之一。由於急症病人之醫療處置上常常充滿不確定性，且急症病人病程演變成重症病人之機率也較其他科別為高，所以與他科醫師間之團隊合作也相對重要。如本案病人，到院時只是中度肺炎，可是在短短一天內病程卻急速惡化，可知一般的胸腔或感染科病房已不再是適合照顧病人之單位；所以我們照會胸腔內科醫師，一方面可以安排病人在離開急診時能住進適合處理此時嚴重病情之胸腔內科加護病房；另一方面可尋求胸腔內科醫師之專業意見，討論是否需在治療上做其他調整，以便更全面地處理、掌握病人之病況，為病人謀求最大之利益。

Consultation Reply Sheet

Name: ○○○　　　Chart Number: ×××××　　　Sex: Male　　　Age : 57

Bed No: ED OBS ××

Dear Dr. ○○○,

　　This 57 year-old man came to our ED on 2023/3/26 due to productive cough for 2 days with fever for 1 day. Augmentin was started initially under the impression of pneumonia. Unfortunately, progressive shortness of breath was noted today. We were consulted for ICU admission.

P.E.:

1. BT: 38.5℃, HR: 118 beats/min, RR: 22 breaths/min, BP: 86/55 mmHg, SpO_2: 92% (O_2 cannula 5 L/min).
2. General Appearance: Acutely ill-looking.
3. Consciousness: Alert and orientated.
4. Chest: Crackles over bilateral lower lungs.

Lab.:

1. WBC 15,600/mm^3 with Seg 93.1%.
2. Finger stick blood sugar a.c / p.c. → 122/168 mg/dL.
3. Sputum culture (2023/3/26) *K.P* sensitive to Ceftriaxone.

Image:

　　CXR follow-up showed pneumonia in progression.

Impression:

1. Pneumonia (*K.P*) with septic shock.
2. Diabetes mellitus.

Plan:

1. Close monitoring of vital sign.
2. Keep Ceftriaxone for pneumonia.
3. Keep aggressive fluid resuscitation and O_2.
4. Intubation PRN.
5. We will arrange ICU bed for this patient.

   Thanks for your consultation.

Chest physician: ○○○

2023/03/27 09:03

結　論

　　以上就是一般常見之急診病歷的閱讀重點，當然，每家醫院會因為各自系統之不同而在病歷格式或作業模式上略有差異，然而只要能掌握這些閱讀病歷及急診處置流程之觀念，加以練習，定能駕輕就熟，事半功倍。

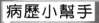

病歷小幫手

Little Helper

　　這是胸腔內科醫師之會診回覆單，回覆之方式仍然依照 SOAP 來進行。第一段簡要說明病人來急診求診之主要問題（咳嗽併發燒）、病人之初步診斷為何（肺炎）、做了什麼處置（給抗生素）、為何現在被照會？（因病情惡化，需要轉入加護病房照顧）。

　　接下來記錄觀察到之病人狀況，包括不穩定之生命徵象及身體檢查不正常之處（肺有爆裂音），再加上白血球偏高，X 光顯示肺炎在惡化，所以做出與急診醫師一致的臆測，即病人之肺炎已進展至敗血性休克，所以在處置方面，除了積極復甦、更換更加強效之抗生素外，也同意要安排胸腔內科加護病房繼續進一步之照顧。

　　當然，並非每次會診他科醫師都會與急診科醫師持相同意見，假如被會診之醫師認為有可能是其他原因造成病況惡化的話，此時也會在會診單上提出其專業看法，這時急診科醫師就必須發揮其整合之能力，居中協調不同科別醫師之意見，為病人謀求最大之福祉。

　　病人最後順利被轉至加護病房，注意急診病人經處置後皆要註明動向，所以病人離開急診時之動向該為 Admission to Chest ICU Bed No. ××；即住入胸腔內科加護病房第××床。

護理小幫手

Little Helper

　　肺炎常見於老年人及慢性病末期病人，常因致病菌大量、快速繁殖，而造成敗血症、敗血性休克、多重器官衰竭等情形，是國人十大死亡原因之一。在病人住院期間，提供的護理措施包括：
1. 依醫囑使用 4~6 L/min 氧氣治療，並需注意缺氧及高碳酸血症的徵象。
2. 痰多時，可利用胸腔物理治療，並教導正確深呼吸及有效咳嗽等方法，以助肺擴張，並促痰咳出。
3. 避免增加氧氣需求的情況，如抽菸及壓力過大。
4. 採高熱量、高蛋白飲食，避免刺激性飲食，並維持 2,000~3,000 c.c.充分的水分攝取，以助稀釋痰液。
5. 多休息及適當的運動（急性期採絕對臥床，恢復期則採漸進性活動）。

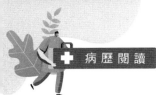
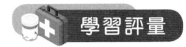

一、選擇題

(　　)1. 有關病人到急診時現病史中之敘述，何者為非？(A)Cough and runny nose for 1 week.　(B)Yellowish sputum noted for 2 days.　(C)Dysuria since last night.　(D)Fever for 1 day.

(　　)2. 急診醫師對於病人在急診觀察室病情惡化時所做之處置，何者為非？(A)Change antibiotic to Ceftriaxone.　(B)Fluid resuscitation.　(C)On foley for fluid status monitoring.　(D)Follow-up Chest X-ray.

(　　)3. 下列何者並非為病人注射中心靜脈導管之過程敘述?(A)The patient was lying in a supine position.　(B)After general anesthesia, central line was inserted smoothly.　(C)The patient was able to tolerate the procedure well without complication.　(D)Follow-up CXR showed that the central line was in an acceptable position.

(　　)4. 有關胸腔內科醫師會診回覆單的建議，何者正確？(A)Keep Augmentin for pneumonia.　(B)Keep aggressive fluid resuscitation and O$_2$.　(C)Intubation immediately.　(D)Arrange chest ward for patient.

(　　)5. 下列何者病人痰液細菌培養所產生之菌種？(A)*Pseudomonas aeruginosa* (B)*Streptococcus pneumoniae*　(C)*Haemophilus influenzae*　(D)*Klebsiella pneumoniae*

二、配合題

( )1. Triage   (A)喘鳴聲

( )2. Shortness of breath   (B)呼吸困難

( )3. Diabetes mellitus   (C)敗血性休克

( )4. Wheezing   (D)革蘭氏染色

( )5. Resuscitation   (E)糖尿病

( )6. Gram stain   (F)血氧分析

( )7. Septic shock   (G)檢傷分類

( )8. Admission   (H)發病危通知

( )9. Blood gas analysis   (I)住院

( )10. On critical condition   (J)復甦

三、填充題

請寫出以下縮寫或生字之全文或中譯。

1. Orthopnea _____

2. PND _____

3. Palpitation _____

4. Bilateral basal crackles _____

5. Hepatosplenomegaly _____

6. Put on central line _____

7. Right internal jugular vein _____

8. Medication _____

9. Consultation Sheet _____

10. Hyperglycemia _____

學習評量解答
請掃描 QR Code

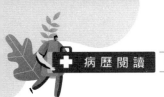
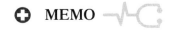
MEMO

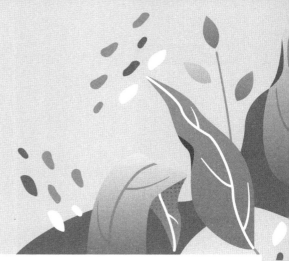

08 | CHAPTER

腫瘤科病歷

作者｜王守玉、卓淑美

Admission Note

Progress Note

Order Sheet

Discharge Summary

☑ **閱讀導引**

1. 了解病人主訴與現在病史的關係。

2. 分析現在病史與過去病史之關聯性。

3. 分析現在病史、檢驗值與治療措施的合適性。

☑ **PREVIEW**

閱讀本章前，請讀者先自行預習腫瘤疾病相關知識喔！

1. 肺癌的血液腫瘤指標有哪些？

2. 肺癌的治療方法。

3. 化學治療的方法與副作用。

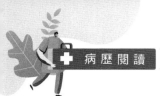
Admission Note

Medical Oncology, Male, 62 years old, Taipei, retired.

Source of information: The patient.

Chief Complaint:

The patient was examined, found to have lung cancer, and was then transferred to our OPD. He experienced **hoarseness** for 5 months before the examination. He is admitted for scheduled **chemotherapy** this time.

Present Illness:

This is a 62 year-old male. According to his statements, he experienced hoarseness for 5 months and was a heavy smoker. Meanwhile, he expressed complaints about vocal palsy during the recent 3 months. In light of the above, he was brought to have a health examination and was then transferred to our OPD for help and a CT arrangement. The CT revealed a lung tumor, which was **adenosquamous** cancer located at the **RLL** with clinical staging of T2bN3M0, stage IIIB. A Port-A catheter was placed via his L't external jugular vein on 2022-8-19.

After his previous chemotherapy, there was no fever, nausea/vomiting nor diarrhea. Under the impression of lung cancer, adenosquamous cancer, RLL, he was admitted for scheduled chemotherapy.

Past History:

This 62 year-old man has a history of hypertension for two years. He is under regular medication.

Personal History:

Way of admission: Walking.　　　Source of admission: OPD.

Education level: Primary school.　Language: Mandarin and Taiwanese.

Marital status: Married.　　　　Children: One son and one daughter.

Living with family.

Occupation: No (retired).

Smoking history: 0.5 pack/day for 40 years.

Drinking history: Yes (1~2 glasses), QOD for 40 years.

Betel nuts chewing: (-).

Travel history for the past month: (-).

Religion: Folk belief.

Family History:

Father: Not contributory.

Mother: Not contributory.

Review of Systems:

1. General: Recent weight change(-), fever or chills(-), decreased appetite(+), fatigue(+), generalized weakness(+), trouble sleeping(-).

2. Skin: Rashes(-), lumps(-), itching(-), dryness(-), color changes(-), hair or nail changes(-).

3. Head & Neck: Headache(-), head injury(-), neck lumps(-), neck stiffness(-), swollen glands(-), neck pain(-).

4. Eyes: Blurred vision(-), double vision(-), redness(-), glaucoma(-), cataracts(-).

5. ENT: Nothing in particular.

6. Breasts: Nothing in particular.

7. Respiratory: Cough(-), sputum(-), hemoptysis(-), shortness of breath(-), wheezing(-), painful breathing(-).

8. Cardiovascular: Chest pain or tightness(-), dyspnea on exertion(-), orthopnea(-), palpitations(-), edema(-), calf pain with walking(-).

9. Gastrointestinal: Swallowing difficulties(-), heartburn(-), decreased appetite(-), nausea and/or vomiting(-), hematemesis(-), melena(-), abdominal pain(-), constipation(-), diarrhea(-), rectal bleeding(-), yellow eyes or skin(-).

10. Urinary: Frequency(-), urgency(-), burning or pain(-), hesitancy(-), blood in urine(-), incontinence(-), nocturia(-), increased urine amount(-), decreased urine amount(-).

11. Genitoreproductive, Male: Nothing in particular..

12. Musculoskeletal: Joint pain(-), stiffness of joints(-), redness of joints(-), swelling of joints (-), limited range of motion(-), myalgia(-), muscle cramp(-), muscle weakness(-), muscle atrophy(-), back pain(-), lumps(-).

13. Neurologic: Dizziness(-), fainting(-), seizure(-), focal weakness(-), numbness or tingling(-), tremor(-).

14. Hematologic: Nothing in particular.

15. Endocrine: Nothing in particular.

16. Psychiatric: Nothing in particular.

Physical Examinations:

1. Vital Signs: T: 37.3°C, P: 97/min, R: 22/min, BP: 125/65 mmHg.

2. BH: 165 cm, BW: 48.8 kg, BMI: 17.9.

3. General Appearance: Consciousness: Alert; oriented to person, place and time; GCS: E4V5M6; nourishment and development: normal; personal hygiene: proper; ill-looking(-).

4. Skin: Cyanosis(-), pallor(-), yellow discoloration(-), **petechia/ecchymosis**(-), rashes(-), swelling/edema(-), specific lesions(-).

5. Lymph nodes: Neck(-), axillary(-), inguinal(-).

6. Head & Neck: Deformity(-), trauma(-), neck stiffness(-), bruit(-), jugular vein engorgement(-), goiter(-), palpable mass(-), specific lesions(-).

7. Eyes: Conjunctiva(-), pale(-), watery eyes(-), sclera: icteric.

8. ENT: Hearing: Normal, nasal lesion(-), oral lesion(-).

9. Chest:
- Thoracic cage: Deformity(-).
- Respiratory pattern: Use of accessory muscles/ retraction(-), **tachypnea**(-).
- Breath sound: Clear and symmetric.

10. Breast: Lump(-), skin dimpling(-), nipple discharge(-).

11. Heart: Rhythm: Regular heart beats, murmurs(-).

12. Abdomen:
- Inspection: Flat; operation scar(-).
- Palpation/percussion: Soft; rigidity/muscle guarding(-), tenderness(-), rebound tenderness (-), shifting dullness(-).
- Auscultation: Bowel sound(-). normoactive; high-pitched bowel sound(-), bruits(-).
- Abnormal signs: Murphy's sign(-), Rovsing's sign(-), iliopsoas sign (-), obturator sign (-).

13. Extremities: Tenderness(-), deformity(-), edema(-).

14. Joints: Tenderness(-), inflammation(-), deformity(-), range of motion: full.

15. Spine: Deformity(-), tenderness(-), knocking pain(-).

16. Specific Findings: Nil.

關鍵字彙 Keywords

字　彙	原　文	中　譯
Hoarseness		聲音嘶啞
Chemotherapy		化學治療
Adenosquamous		腺性鱗狀上皮細胞
RLL	right lower lobe	右下肺葉
Petechia		紫斑
Ecchymosis		瘀斑
Tachypnea		呼吸急促

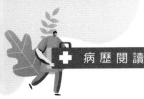
Laboratory:

1. CBC

Date	WBC	RBC	Hb	Hct	MCV	PLT	Basophils	Monocytes	Neutrophils
2023/02/04	3,700 uL	2.58*10⁶ uL	8.8 g/dL	26.3 %	102 fL	234,000 uL	1.0 %	14.0 %	30.0 %

2. BCS

Date	Glocuse AC	BUN	Creatinine	AST	ALK-P	Albumin	Sodium	Potassium	Chloride
2023/02/04	97 mg/dL	17 mg/dL	1.0 mg/dL	17 U/L	62 U/L	3.7 g/dL	138 mEq/L	3.7 mEq/L	101 mEq/L

護理小幫手　　　　　　　　　　　　　　　　　　　　　　Little Helper

腹部檢查中相關的測試

* Murphy's sign (+)：膽囊炎
* Rovsing's sign (+)：闌尾炎
* Iliopsoas sign (+)：闌尾炎
* McBurney's sign (+)：闌尾炎

資料來源：Fenske, C., Watkins, K., Saunders, T., D'Amico, D., & Barbarito, C. (2022)．*健康與身體檢查*（二版）（蔡佩珊等譯）．華杏。（原著出版於 2019）

護理小幫手　　　　　　　　　　　　　　　　　　　　　　Little Helper

血液檢驗

　　Neutrophil：相對值 45~75%，絕對值 2,000~7,500/μL，當其減少時，常見於病人有慢性感染、病毒性感染、自體免疫或末梢之血球破壞等；當絕對值小於 500 μL，容易受到黴菌及細菌的感染。

　　化學治療藥物是利用對於身體生長較快的細胞影響較大，來達到抑制癌細胞的目的，但通常，除了腫瘤細胞外，其他生長快速的細胞也易受影響。骨髓是身體內主要的造血組織，所以化療後幾乎都會產生某種程度的「骨髓抑制」，而引起白血球、紅血球及血小板數目降低的副作用。醫師會評估病人的狀況，再決定此次是否可進行化療，或是以降低劑量的方式進行治療。

資料來源：王嘉莉、王德珍、王繁棻、朱繼璋、余文瑞、李隆乾、周玉蘭、林志遠、林佩菁、林季榆、洪淑萍、胡逸然、張勝雄、郭佩勳、陳富鈞、陳燕彰、陳證文、曾偉誠、曾梓維…顏永豐(2017)．於楊文理主編，*臨床檢驗判讀*（二版）．新文京。

護理小幫手

腫瘤的分期 Staging

TNM 分期系統

T：原發性腫瘤，侵蝕深度、大小

TX：無法評估原發腫瘤

T0：原發部位無腫瘤證據

TIS：癌細胞僅在表層組織，未侵犯到深層組織，又稱原位癌(carcinoma in situ, CIS)

T1-T4：腫瘤大小及散播的範圍，T 的數字越高，侵蝕程度越大

N：癌細胞是否侵犯附近的淋巴結

NX：局部淋巴結無法被評估

N0：淋巴結無癌細胞

N1-N3：癌細胞侵犯淋巴結的大小、範圍及數量，N 的數字越高，侵蝕程度越大

M：癌細胞是否有遠端轉移

M0：沒有遠端轉移

M1：有遠端轉移到器官或組織

根據 TNM 分期系統，可分為 0-IV 期，其中又可細分 IIA、IIB、IIIA、IIIB：

Stage 0：原位癌，需做局部切除

Stage I：腫瘤局限於原發組織，無侵犯淋巴結及遠端轉移

Stage II：腫瘤已侵蝕附近的組織及淋巴結，但無遠端轉移

Stage III：腫瘤變更大，已侵蝕更深層的組織及淋巴結

Stage IV：腫瘤變更大，已侵蝕更深層的組織及淋巴結並有遠端轉移

資料來源： American Cancer Society. (2015, Jul 4). *Staging*. http://www.cancer.org/treatment/understandingyourdiagnosis/staging

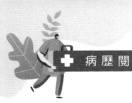
Radiology & Imaging Reports:

Chest 1 view

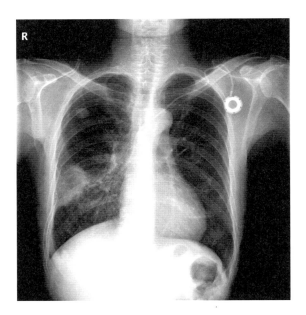

Follow up film of the chest PA view shows a mass in the Rt. Lower lung field and a nodule in the Rt. Upper lung field that is smaller in size compared to the previous film dated Dec. 10, 2022. There is a **port-A line insertion** in the left upper thorax and with mild prominence of the aortic knob noted.

Impression:

Malignant neoplasm of bronchus and lung.

Diagnostic Plans:

1. Follow up CXR, CBC and biochemistry.
2. Check **tumor marker** such as CEA and SCC.

Therapeutic Plans:

1. Chemotherapy with navelbine + CDDP if effective.
2. Prevent side effect related to chemotherapy.

3. Ongoing **R/T**.

4. Supportive medication.

Educational Plans:

1. Educate side effects of chemotherapy.

2. Explain the current clinical condition to the patient and his family, and follow up the treatment directions.

Attending Physician: ×××

Resident: △△△

 Thinking About ////////////////////////////

1. 何謂 Port-A？為何病人要 on Port-A？

2. 何謂 CEA, SCC？為何病人要追蹤 CEA, SCC？

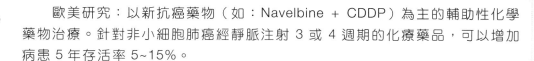

護理小幫手

Little Helper

　　歐美研究：以新抗癌藥物（如：Navelbine + CDDP）為主的輔助性化學藥物治療。針對非小細胞肺癌經靜脈注射 3 或 4 週期的化療藥品，可以增加病患 5 年存活率 5~15%。

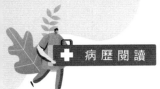

Progress Note

Medical Oncology, Male, 62 years old, Taipei, retired.

Date of admission: 2023-02-04.

2023-2-5

#1 Local advanced lung cancer, stage IIIB

S:

1. Fair appetite.
2. No fever.

O:

1. General: fair-looking, conscious: alert.
2. Vital signs: T: 36°C, P: 93/min, R: 19/min, BP: 132/67 mmHg.
3. Chest: Symmetric expansion, clear breathing sounds; regular heart beat, no murmur.
4. Abdomen: Soft and flat; percussion: dullness; normoactive bowel sound, no **epigastralgia**.
5. Lower extremity: Warm, no pitting edema, freely movable.
6. Skin: No skin turgor.

A:

1. Locally advanced lung cancer, stage IIIB.
2. Arrange chemotherapy today (Vinorelbine + Cisplatin on 2023-02-05).

P:

1. Arrange chemotherapy today (Vinorelbine + Cisplatin on 2023-02-05).
2. Educate him on side effects of chemotherapy.
3. **Symptomatic** treatment.
4. Keep OPD treatment.
5. Close observation of vital signs.
6. Explain the current clinical condition to the patient and his family, and follow up the treatment directions.

Attending Physician: ✕✕✕

Resident: △△△

關鍵字彙 Keywords

字　彙	原　文	中　譯
Port-A line insertion		人工血管植入
Malignant		惡性的
Neoplasm		贅生物
Tumor marker		腫瘤標記
R/T	radiotherapy	放射治療
Epigastralgia		上腹痛
Symptomatic		症狀的

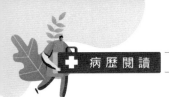

Order Sheet

Medical Oncology Male, 62 years old, Taipei, retired.

Date of admission: 2023-02-04.

Chemotherapy Order

Diagnosis: Malignant neoplasm of bronchus and lung.

Regimen: Vinorelbine (60)-PO + Cisplatin (60)-N/S 1,000   Course: **C**6**D**8

Path: Port-A.

BH: 165 cm   BW: 49 kg   **BSA**: 1.5 m^2 **CCR**: 45.37   **PS**: 1.

Chemotherapy permission: OK.

2023-02-05 08:50:23

#Pre-medication

1. Metoclopramide (10 mg/ 2mL amp) 1 ampoule IV STAT on 02/05 before chemotherapy.

2. Dexamethasone phosphate/Dexamethasone (5 mg/ 1mL amp) ampoule IV STAT on 02/05 before chemotherapy.

3. Granisetron (3 mg/3 mL vial) 1 vial + Sodium chloride 0.9% (20 mL amp) 15 c.c. IVD run 15 mins STAT on 02/05 before chemotherapy.

4. Sodium chloride 0.9%/ (500 mL bot) 500 c.c. IVD run 3 hours STAT on 02/05.

【Before Cisplatin】

#Chemotherapy

1. Cisplatin 92 mg (60 MG/m^2) (102.222% dose) in Sodium chloride 0.9% (500 mL bot) 1,000 c.c. IVD running 10 hours on 02/05.

2. Vinorelbine 5 cap (60 MG/m^2) (5.555% dose) PO on 02/05.

#<u>Adjuvant</u>

1. Metoclopramide (10 mg/2 mL amp) 1 ampoule Q8H IV on 02/05, 02/06.

2. Dexamethasone phosphate/Dexamethasone (5 mg/1 mL amp) 1 ampoule Q8H IV on 02/05, 02/06.

3. Furosemide 1 ampoule IV STAT on 02/06.

【after post-cisplatin <u>hydration</u>】

4. Sodium chloride 0.9% (500 mL bot) 500 c.c. IVD run 3 hours STAT on 02/06.

【post Cisplatin】

 關鍵字彙 Keywords

字　彙	原　文	中　譯
C	course	療程
D	day	天
BSA	body surface area	體表面積
CCR	creatinine clearance rate	肌酐酸廓清率
PS	performance status	日常體能狀態
Adjuvant		輔助藥物
Hydration		補水（水合作用）

Thinking About

1. 化學治療前、後為什麼要補充點滴輸液？
2. 化學治療有何作用及副作用？
3. 化學治療前為什麼要先給止吐及類固醇藥物？
4. 除了化學治療需要算體表面積之外，還有哪些治療需要用到體表面積？
5. 此類的病人做完化學治療或放射線治療回家後需注意什麼？

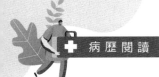

護理小幫手

Little Helper

　　肺癌的全身性治療，包括化學治療及標靶治療。肺癌可分為小細胞肺癌及非小細胞肺癌。整體而言，非小細胞肺癌的預後比小細胞肺癌來得好。

　　腺鱗狀癌屬於非小細胞肺癌，其化學治療分為兩類：一種是第二或第三期的病人，於手術後，需要給予輔助性化學治療，以降低復發的機率，這時藥物的標準選項為 Vinorelbine 合併 Cisplatin。一般 Cisplatin 大約都是 21 天的週期，第一週期跟第二週期的劑量與注射時間會不一樣，如果沒有特殊反應，注射時間與劑量就會固定下來。

　　另一種情況是無法手術的晚期病人，根據臨床上的研究顯示，接受化學治療的病人比沒有接受化學治療的病人活得久，而且生活品質也可維持於較好的情況。

資料來源：和信治癌中心醫院（2017，5 月 11 日）·*精確醫療(precision medicine)：正確使用藥物才是肺癌個人化醫療的適當方向*。http://www.kfsyscc.org/cancer/lung-cancer/guideline/med/

Discharge Summary

Admission Diagnosis:

#1. Lung Ca. (adenosquamous ca., RLL, T2bN3M0, stage IIIB) with vocal palsy s/p C/T (Vinorelbine + Cisplatin on 2023-01-09).

#2. Essential hypertension.

#3. Right chest pain.

Discharge Diagnosis:

1. Lung Ca. (adenosquamous ca., RLL, T2bN3M0, stage IIIB) with vocal palsy s/p C/T (Vinorelbine + Cisplatin on 2023-02-05).

2. Essential hypertension.

Chief Complaint:

Intermittent right side chest pain for two days.

Brief History:

This 62 year-old man has histories of: 1. Lung Ca. (adenosquamous ca., RLL, T2bN3M0, stage IIIB) with vocal palsy s/p C/T (Vinorelbine + Cisplatin on 2023-01-09) 2. Essential hypertension presented with intermittent right side chest pain for two days.

Lung Ca. (adenosquamous ca., RLL, T2bN3M0, stage IIIB) was diagnosed with initial presentation of hoarseness and vocal palsy for months. Port-A catheter was placed via his L't external jugular vein on 2022-8-19.

After the last chemotherapy, there has been no fever, nausea/vomiting nor diarrhea. Schedule chemotherapy was arranged this time. However, he complained about right chest pain with exacerbation. There were no fever, SOB, nor cold sweating, but with only a mild cough mentioned. Chest PA view showed a round mass lesion at the right lower lung with one **nodular** **lesion** at the right upper lung. There was no significant change in compared to the last chest film, in which the Port-A catheter insertion was also seen.

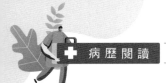
Under the impression of right chest pain, favor lung cancer related, he was admitted for further evaluation and management.

Review of Systems:

1. General: Recent weight change(-), fever or chills(-), decreased appetite(-), fatigue(+), generalized weakness(+), trouble sleeping(-).

2. Skin: Rashes(-), lumps(-), itching(-), dryness(-), color changes(-), hair or nail changes(-).

3. Head & Neck: Headache(-), head injury(-), neck lumps(-), neck stiffness(-), swollen glands　(-), neck pain(-).

4. Eyes: Blurred vision(-), double vision(-), redness(-), glaucoma(-), cataracts(-).

5. ENT: Nothing in particular.

6. Breasts: Nothing in particular.

7. Respiratory: Cough(-), sputum(-), hemoptysis(-), shortness of breath(-), wheezing(-), painful breathing(-).

8. Cardiovascular: Chest pain or tightness(-), dyspnea on exertion(-), orthopnea(-), palpitations (-), edema(-), calf pain with walking(-).

9. Gastrointestinal: Swallowing difficulties(-), heartburn(-), decreased appetite(-), nausea and/or vomiting(-), hematemesis(-), melena(-), abdominal pain(-), constipation(-), diarrhea(-), rectal bleeding(-), yellow eyes or skin(-).

10. Urinary: Frequency(-), urgency(-), burning or pain(-), hesitancy(-), blood in urine(-), incontinence(-), nocturia(-), increased urine amount(-), decreased urine amount(-).

11. Genitoreproductive, Male: Nothing in particular.

12. Musculoskeletal: Joint pain(-), stiffness of joints(-), redness of joints(-), swelling of joints(-), limited range of motion(-), myalgia(-), muscle cramp(-), muscle weakness(-), muscle atrophy(-), back pain(-), lumps (-).

13. Neurologic: Dizziness(-), fainting(-), seizures(-), focal weakness(-), numbness or tingling(-), tremor(-).

14. Hematologic: Nothing in particular.

15. Endocrine: Nothing in particular.

16. Psychiatric: Nothing in particular.

Physical Examinations:

1. Vital Signs: T: 37.6°C, P: 100/min, R: 20/min, BP: 142/78 mmHg.

2. BH: 161 cm, BW: 53.2 kg, BMI: 20.5.

3. General Appearance: Consciousness: Alert; GCS: E4V5M6; **Ill-looking**(+).

4. Skin: Pallor(-).

5. Head and Neck: Palpable mass(-).

6. ENT: Others: Hoarseness and vocal palsy.

7. Chest:
   - Breath sounds: Diminished breath sounds(+), at right lung.
   - Others: Intermittent right side chest pain.

8. Heart: Murmurs(-).

9. Abdomen:
   - Inspection: Flat.
   - Palpation/percussion: Soft.
   - Auscultation: Bowel sound: Normoactive.

10. Rectal exam: Normal rectal sphincter tone(-), Anal fistula(-).

11. External genitalia-Male.
   - Prostate: Warts: (+).

12. Extremities: Tenderness(-), Deformity(-).

13. Neurological exam: Cranial nerves I-XII: Normal.

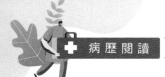

Laboratory:

1. CBC

Date	WBC	RBC	Hb	Hct	MCV	PLT	Basophils	Monocytes	Neutrophils
2023/02/05	4,200 uL	$2.58*10^6$ uL	9.2 g/dL	26.3 %	100 fL	250,000 uL	1.0 %	15.0 %	50.0 %

2. BCS

Date	Glocuse AC	BUN	Creatinine	AST	ALK-P	Albumin	Sodium	Potassium	Chloride
2023/02/05	100 mg/dL	17 mg/dL	1.1 mg/dL	17 U/L	75 U/L	3.9 g/dL	140 mEq/L	4.2 mEq/L	105 mEq/L

Course and Treatment:

This time, he was admitted to our ward for a course of chemotherapy and right chest pain. After admission, chemotherapy was performed smoothly (Vinorelbine (60 mg)-PO + Cisplatin (60 mg)-N/S 1,000 c.c.). During the chemotherapy, there was no fever, chillness, headache, dizziness, cough with **yellowish sputum**, sore throat, nausea, vomiting, chest discomfort, abdominal tenderness, urinary frequency/urgency, diarrhea/constipation, muscle soreness, skin rash, nor any other allergic reaction. According to the relatively stable vital signs, fair **appetite**, normal activity, and stable condition, he was discharged from our ward today with a further OPD follow up arranged.

Complication:

Nil.

Status on Discharge:

Stable.

Recommendations & Medications:

OPD follow up.

Attending Physician: ×××

Resident: △△△

關鍵字彙 Keywords

字 彙	中 譯
Nodular	小結節
Lesion	損傷
Ill-looking	病態倦容
Yellowish sputum	黃痰
Appetite	食慾

護理小幫手

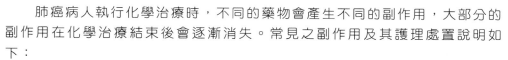

Little Helper

　　肺癌病人執行化學治療時，不同的藥物會產生不同的副作用，大部分的副作用在化學治療結束後會逐漸消失。常見之副作用及其護理處置說明如下：

1. 噁心嘔吐：採少量多餐的清淡飲食，可利用聽音樂、看書轉移注意力或穴位按壓。嘔吐後注意口腔清潔。
2. 血球減少：可能導致感染、貧血及出血現象。需觀察瘀斑、出血情形，避免受傷或感染、不要接觸已知有感染的人，以及經常洗手、維持良好衛生習慣。改變姿勢時，動作需緩慢，以免頭暈而跌倒。
3. 口腔潰瘍：維持口腔衛生，鼓勵口腔乾燥時多喝水，並避免粗糙或刺激性食物。
4. 掉髮：衛教病人掉髮是暫時性，可預先減短頭髮，並建議可選購合適的假髮、帽子、頭巾。
5. 疲憊：需充足的休息及適當的運動。可局部的按摩，促進血液循環，增加舒適。

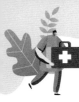

學習評量

一、選擇題

(　　)1. 以下何者是病人主要的入院診斷？(A)HIVD　(B)Type 2 DM　(C)Hepatoma (D)Lung cancer

(　　)2. 請問病人的個人病史中下列何者為是？(A)病人由急診入院　(B)病人有菸癮 40 年　(C)病人單身　(D)病人過去一個月曾出國旅遊

(　　)3. Decreased appetite 的中譯為何？(A)食慾降低　(B)食慾提高　(C)活動力降 低　(D)活動力提高

(　　)4. 病人的系統性評估與身體檢查方面，下列何者為是？(A)病人有暈眩的情形 (B)病人的 Murphy's sign(+)　(C)病人有發燒情形　(D)病人有全身虛弱的情 形

(　　)5. 下列何項為類固醇類的藥物？(A)Cisplatin　(B)Dexamethasone (C)Furosemide　(D)Granisetron

二、配合題

(　　)1.　Hoarseness

(　　)2.　Petechia

(　　)3.　Tachypnea

(　　)4.　Folk belief

(　　)5.　Tumor marker

(　　)6.　Port-A line insertion

(　　)7.　Malignant

(　　)8.　CCR

(　　)9.　Nodular

(　　)10. Ill-looking

(A)腫瘤標記

(B)低血鉀

(C)肝性腦病變

(D)中心靜脈導管（人工 血管）植入

(E)腎絲球腎炎

(F)惡性的

(G)聲音沙啞

(H)手腳麻痺

(I)呼吸急促

(J)尿素氮

(K)血液肌酸酐廓清試驗

(L)民間信仰

(M)肌酸酐

(N)病態倦容

(O)小結節

(P)紫斑

(Q)良性

(R)淋巴結

(S)吞嚥困難

(T)僵直

三、填充題

請寫出以下縮寫或生字之全文及中譯。

1. Chemotherapy _____

2. Radiotherapy _____

3. Aortic knob _____

4. External jugular vein _____

5. Essential hypertension _____

6. Yellowish sputum _____

7. Seizures _____

8. Swelling/edema _____

9. Extremities _____

10. Adenosquamous _____

學習評量解答
請掃描 QR Code

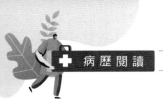
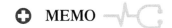

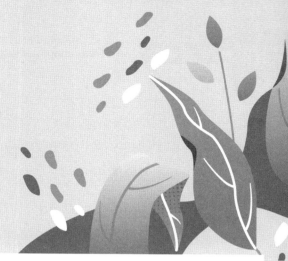

09 | CHAPTER

牙科病歷

作者｜李正喆、魏鈴穎

Admission Note

Progress Note

Order Sheet

Discharge Summary

☑ **閱讀導引**

1. 了解病人主訴與現在病史的關係。
2. 分析現在病史與過去病史之關聯性。
3. 分析現在病史、檢驗值與治療措施的合適性。

☑ **PREVIEW**

閱讀本章前，請讀者先自行預習蜂窩性組織炎相關知識喔！

1. 蜂窩性組織炎的臨床表徵？
2. 頭頸部感染的組織間隙有哪些？
3. 牙科齒位記錄法（內有附圖）

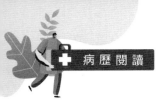

Admission Note

Dentistry, Male, 18 years old, Taipei, college student.

Source of information: The patient.

Identifying information:

Name: XXX   Chart Number: 5546677.

Gender: Male   Age: 18.

Occupation: College student.

Chief Complaint:

Evaluation of painful facial swelling and limitation of mouth opening.

Present Illness:

This 18 year-old male complained of **gum** swelling at his lower left posterior teeth and **progression** of facial swelling for 7 days. In these days, he had episodes of fever. He went to local dental clinic for help, and took some antibiotics and painkillers before coming to our outpatient department. However, the pain persisted, and the **lip numbness** occurred, which alarmed the patient to seek for further treatment.

Past Medical History:

1. Systemic diseases: Asthma, under control with steroid.

2. Surgical history: Denied.

3. Travel history: Denied in the past 6 months.

4. Current medication:

   (1) NTUH: Nil.

   (2) Others: Amolin (250 mg) 1# Q8H, Paramol (500 mg) 1# QID.

Past Dental History:

1. **Dental restoration**(+).

2. **Endodontic treatment**(-).

3. **Dental extraction**(-).

4. **Dental prosthesis**(-).

5. **Scaling** was performed 3 months ago.

Personal History:

1. Alcohol consumption: Denied.

2. Smoking: 0.5 PPD (pack per day), for 2 years.

3. Betel quid chewing: Denied.

4. Drug allergy history: Ibuprofen, Ponstan.

Local Finding:

1. Extraoral findings:

- **Trismus**, with **maximum mouth opening** (MMO): 8 mm, with bilateral muscle tenderness.
- Left facial swelling, involving left buccal and submandibular space.
  - Local heat (+).
  - Skin redness (+).
  - Consistency: Firm.
- A reactive lymph node was palpable in the left level Ib of neck.
  - Size: 1 cm in diameter.
  - Mobility: Movable, not fixed.
  - Consistency: Elastic.
  - Tenderness: Mild.

Dental Numbering Systems
(Permanent Teeth)

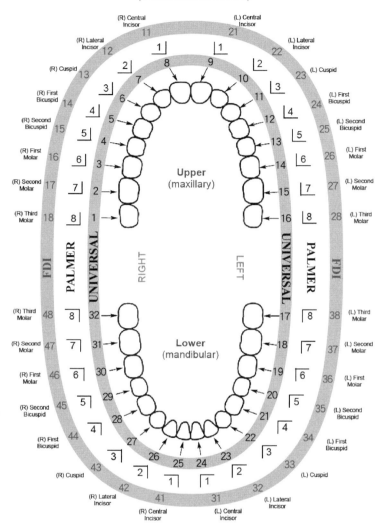

2. Intraoral findings:

- #36-#38 buccal **gingival swelling** was noted.
- Buccal **vestibule elevation**, with **fluctuation**.
- A **partial erupted** #38 was noticed.
- Palpation and percussion pain (+).
- No visible **dental caries** in the region.

3. Panoramic X-ray findings:

- A mesioangulated #38 was <u>impacted</u> > it may be the <u>offending tooth</u>.
- The root formation of #38 is not complete.

4. Periapical X-ray findings:

- Radiolucency around crown portion of #38.
- No detectable caries.

Family History:

DM (+): Patient's father.

Review of Systems:

1. Systemic: Weight loss(-), easy-fatigability(+), night sweats(-).

2. Skin: Petechiae(-), purpura(-), skin rash(+), itching(-).

3. HEENT: Headache(-), dizziness(-), blurred vision(-), strabismus(-), ocular pain(-), otalgia(-), otorrhea(-), hearing impairment(-), tinnitus(-), vertigo(-), nasal stuffiness(-), nasal discharge (-), epistaxis(-), gum bleeding (+, small amount, intermittent), sore throat(-), oral ulcer(-), cheek swelling with local erythematous change and local heat (+).

4. Cardiovascular: Exertional chest tightness(-), nocturnal dyspnea(-), orthopnea(-), syncope(-), palpitation(-), intermittent claudication(-).

5. Respiratory: Dyspnea(-), cough(-), chest pain(-), hemoptysis(-), productive cough(-), pleuritic chest pain(-).

6. Gastrointestinal: Anorexia(-), nausea(-), vomiting(-), dysphagia(+), heartburn(-), acid regurgitation(-), abdominal fullness(-), hunger pain(-) midnight pain(-), constipation(-), diarrhea(-), melena(-), change of bowel habit(-), small caliber of stool(-), tenesmus(-), flatulence(-).

7. Urogenital: Flank pain(-), hematuria(-), urinary frequency(-), urgency(-), dysuria(-), hesitancy(-), small stream of urine(-), impotence(-), nocturia(-), polyuria(-), oliguria (-).

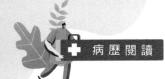

8. Musculoskeletal: Bone pain(-), arthralgia(-), myalgia(-), weakness(-), back pain(-).

9. Metabolic: Heat intolerance(-), cold intolerance(-), thirsty(-).

10. Nervous: Numbness (+, lower lip), paresis/plegia(-).

Physical Examinations:

1. BH: 180 cm, BW: 56 kg.

2. Vital signs: T: 37.5℃, RR: 18/min, HR 86/min, BP: 102/57 mmHg.

3. Pain sore: 6/10.

4. Neurological Examination:
   - Consciousness: Clear, GCS: E4M6V5.
   - Muscle power: Full but mild general malaise.
   - Gait: Steady but weak.

5. HEENT: Cheek swelling with local erythematous change and local heat.

6. Neck:
   - Jugular vein engorgement(-).
   - Thyroid goiter(-).
   - Carotid bruit(-).
   - Lymphadenopathy(+): Left level Ib, 1 cm, rule out reactive lymph node.

7. Heart: Regular heart beat without murmur.

8. Chest: Clear breathing sound.

9. Abdomen: Soft and flat, normoactive bowel sound.

10. Extremities: Freely movable, no edema.

關鍵字彙 Keywords

字　彙	原　文	中　譯
Gum		牙齦，又稱 gingiva
Progression		進展、擴大
Lip Numbness		嘴唇麻木
Dental restoration		補牙
Endodontic treatment		根管治療
Dental extraction		拔牙
Dental prosthesis		假牙
Scaling		洗牙
Trismus		張口困難
MMO	maximum mouth opening	最大張口度
Gingival swelling		牙齦腫
Vestibule elevation		前庭鼓起，指原本應為凹陷處，卻因腫脹而鼓起
Fluctuation		波動感，可能有液體或膿腫蓄積
Partial erupted		部分萌出（的牙齒）
Dental caries		齲齒、蛀牙
Impacted		阻生的、無法萌發的
Offending tooth		引起病症之患齒
Wisdom tooth		智齒

Laboratory:

1. BCS

Date	Glucose	Cr.	BUN	ALT	Sodium	Potassium	Chloride	CRP
2023/3/22	134 mg/dL	0.6 mg/dL	5.4 mg/dL	33 U/L	136 mmol/L	4.2 mmol/L	93 mmol/L	21.45 mg/dL

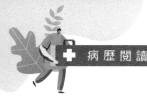
2. CBC

Date	WBC	RBC	Hb	Seg	Band	PLT	Lymphocyte	Monocyte
2023/3/22	23,170/uL	4.77 M/uL	14.3 g/dL	86.7%	0%	599,000/uL	6.0%	7.2%

3. Coagulation

Date	PT	PT cont	PTT	INR
2023/3/22	12.7 sec	11.3 sec	35.7 sec	1.20

護理小幫手

Little Helper

　　大約 90%以上的頭頸部感染是由牙齒的病變所引起，當出現紅腫熱痛、發燒或有張口困難等現象時，需先排除齒源性感染之可能。慢性症狀如皮膚瘻管(skin fistula)或鼻竇炎，亦可能來自齒源性感染，必要時應請牙科醫師或口腔顎面外科醫師診治，頭頸部的蜂窩組織炎或壞死性筋膜炎(necrotizing fasciitis)，極可能成為致命的感染疾病。

　　若齒源性感染未經適當治療，感染即有可能蔓延而造成嚴重的深層頭頸部筋膜間隙感染，若腫脹壓迫到氣管，可能導致呼吸道阻塞或有窒息危險。當兩側之舌下、頜下、頦下間隙同時感染時，稱為 Ludwig 氏咽峽炎(Ludwig's angina)，甚至需要靠緊急氣管切開術來救命，亦可能導致敗血性休克而死亡。或沿咽旁、後咽間隙感染往下蔓延導致胸部中隔腔炎(mediastinitis)。

　　嚴重的深層頭頸部筋膜間隙感染常發生在年紀較大、抵抗力較差或免疫力有缺陷的病人身上，例如控制不良的糖尿病、長期服用類固醇、癌症、洗腎病人。而不良的口腔環境往往是造成感染的主要因素，保持良好的口腔衛生為預防頭頸部齒源性感染的不二法門。

Radiology & Imaging Reports:

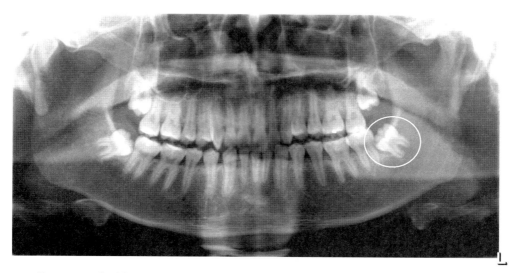

Panoramic X-ray: showed impacted #38 in the offending region

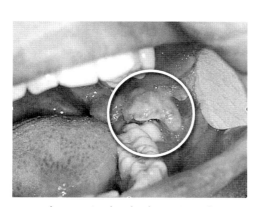

Impacted <u>wisdom tooth</u>

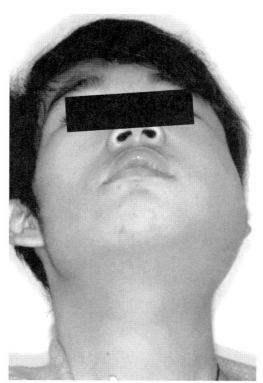

facial swelling

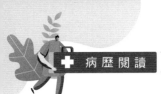

Impression:

1. Facial cellulitis, involving left buccal and submandibular spaces.
2. Offending tooth: impacted #38, with pericoronitis.

Diagnostic Plans:

Head and neck CT with/without contrast: to evaluate the involved spaces and the airway patency.

Therapeutic Plans:

1. Set IV lines for parenteral antibiotics.
2. Extraoral incision and drainage (I&D).

Educational plans:

1. Explain the clinical course of disease and related treatments.
2. Explain the indication, method, risk and complications of operation.

Attending Physician: ×××

Resident: △△△

Progress Note

Dentistry, Male, 18 years old, Taipei, college student.

Date of admission: 2023-03-22.

2023-3-22

#1 <u>Odontogenic</u> cellulitis with abscess formation.

S: fever <u>on and off</u>.

O:

1. T/P/R: 38℃/84 bpm/18 bpm, BP: 121/81 mmHg, VAS: 3.

2. Pain relief under Ultracet and Tramal.

3. Facial swelling: Painful tenderness, no improvement after **parenteral antibiotics** (D3).

4. The H&N CT showed **abscess formation** in the left masticator space, and suspected **osteomyelitis**.

A: **Odontogenic** cellulitis, involving the left buccal, submandibular and masticator spaces.

P:

1. **NPO**, with slow hydration.

2. Preparation for **surgical intervention**.

Attending Physician: ×××

Resident: △△△

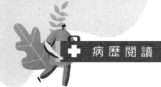

 關鍵字彙 Keywords

字　彙	原　文	中　譯
Odontogenic		齒源性的
On and off		（體溫）忽高忽低
Parenteral antibiotics		靜脈注射抗生素
Abscess formation		形成膿腫
Osteomyelitis		骨髓炎
NPO	*nil per os* (nothing by mouth)	禁食
Surgical intervention		外科手術

Order Sheet

Dentistry, Male, 18 years old, Taipei, college student.

Date of admission: 2023-03-22.

Pre-OP order

2023-3-22

1. Sign the consent and permit.

2. Sent patient to OR at 08:00 tomorrow morning.

3. Regular antibiotic IV push.

Attending Physician: ××××

Resident: △△△

Post-OP order

2023-3-23

1. On 6W3 routine.

2. Set **IVF** N/S 100 mL/hr. (total 500 mL) on **POD1**.

3. N/S irrigation through the **penrose drain** and change dressing Q8H.

4. NG feeding, 2,250 cal/day.

5. Naposin 250 mg 1# TID PC.

6. Keep Unasyn 2,000 mg Q6H and wait for result of bacterial culture.

7. Arrange appointment for #38 extraction after swelling subsides.

Attending Physician: ××××

Resident: △△△

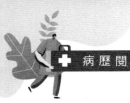

 關鍵字彙 Keywords

字　彙	原　文	中　譯
IVF	intravenous fluid	靜脈輸液
POD1	post-operation day 1	術後第一天
Penrose drain		一種開放式引流管

 Thinking About

1. 當有頭頸部腫脹懷疑是齒源性感染時，可以做哪些檢查？
2. 常見的齒源性感染之菌種為何？適合的經驗性抗生素為何？
3. 一般術前的準備有哪些？
4. 為何要放置引流管？
5. 口腔手術後常見的進食方法？

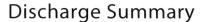

Discharge Summary

Dentistry, Male, 18 years old, Taipei, college student.

Source of information: The patient himself.

Date of admission: 2023-3-22.

Date of discharge: 2023-3-28.

Admission Diagnosis:

1. Deep neck infection with left submandibular space abscess.
2. Offending tooth #38 mesioangular impaction.

Discharge diagnosis:

1. Deep neck infection with left submandibular, submasseteric, parapharyngeal, pterygomandibular space abscess status post operation.
2. Offending tooth #38 mesioangular impaction status post operation.

Chief complaint:

Evaluation of painful facial swelling and limitation of mouth opening.

Brief History:

This 18 year-old male complained of gum swelling at his lower left posterior teeth and progression of facial swelling for 7 days. In these days, he had episodes of fever. He went to local dental clinic for help, and took some antibiotics and painkillers before coming to our outpatient department. However, the pain persisted, and the lip numbness occurred, which alarmed the patient to seek for further treatment. Systemic antibiotics as Unasyn 2g Q6H was initiated. Head and neck CT revealed abscess formation in the left masticator space, and suspected osteomyelitis. Under the impression of deep neck infection, he was admitted for further management.

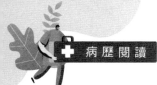

Past History:

1. Systemic diseases: Asthma, under control with steroid.

2. Surgical history: Denied.

3. Travel history: Denied in the past 6 months.

4. Current medication:
   - NTUH: Nil.
   - Others: Amolin (250 mg) 1#Q8H, paramol (500 mg) 1#QID.

Physical Examinations:

1. Physical examination at admission:
   (1) BH: 180 cm, BW: 56 kg.
   (2) T: 37.5, RR: 18, HR 86, BP: 102/57 mmHg, Pain sore: 6/10.

2. Neurological Examination:
   (1) Consciousness: Clear, GCS: E4M6V5.
   (2) Muscle power: Full but mild general malaise.
   (3) Gait: Steady but weak.

3. HEENT: Cheek swelling with local erythematous change and local heat.

4. Neck:
   (1) Jugular vein engorgement (-).
   (2) Thyroid goiter (-).
   (3) Carotid bruit (-).
   (4) Lymphadenopathy (+): left level Ib, 1 cm, rule out reactive lymph node.

5. Heart: Regular heart beat without murmur.

6. Chest: Clear breathing sound.

7. Abdomen: Soft and flat, normoactive bowel sound.

8. Extremities: Freely movable, no edema.

Event Transfer/Discharge change of physical findings:

1. BH: 180 cm, BW: 56 kg.
2. T: 35.8℃, RR: 19/min, HR 89/mon, BP: 122/80 mmHg, Pain sore: 0/10.
3. HEENT:
   (1) left facial swelling subsided, MMO increased from 8 mm to 25 mm.
   (2) dyspnea (-), dysphagia (-).
   (3) wound healing of #38 extraction wound: oozing (-), normal healing.

Operation:

1. Operation date: 2023-3-23.
2. Operation method: Deep neck incision and drainage, debridement.
3. Operation finding:
   (1) Offending tooth: #38 pericoronitis with mesioangular impaction.
   (2) Deep neck infection with left submandibular, submasseteric, parapharyngeal, pterygomandibular space involvement.
   (3) Much purulent discharge at I&D site.

Course and Treatment:

After admission, systemic antibiotics as Unasyn 2g Q6H was initiated. Head and neck CT revealed deep neck infection. The operation of incision and drainage was then held on the next day. After operation, the facial swelling subsided gradually. He was discharged on 2023-03-28.

Complication:

Nil.

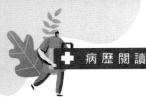
Laboratory:

1. BCS

Date	Glucose	Cre	BUN	ALT	Sodium	Potassium	Chloride	CRP
2023/3/18	134 mg/dL	0.6 mg/dL	5.4 mg/dL	33U/L	136 mmol/L	4.2 mmol/L	93 mmol/L	21.45 mg/dL

2. CBC

Date	WBC	RBC	Hb	Seg	Band	PLT	Lymphocyte	Monocyte
2023/3/18	23,170/uL	4.77 M/uL	14.3 g/dL	86.7%	0%	599,000/uL	6.0%	7.2%

3. Coagulation

Date	PT	PT cont	PTT	INR
2023/3/18	12.7 sec	11.3 sec	35.7 sec	1.20

Imaging Report:

2023-3-22 Chest: PA view (Standing) normal heart size. No active lung lesion.

Pathological Report:

Pending.

Discharge planning:

1. Discharge condition: stable and OPD recall on 2023-4-8.

2. Medication: Ultracet 1# PO QID and Augmentin (1g) 1# BID for 7 days.

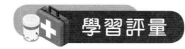 **學習評量**

一、選擇題

( )1. 請問經檢查後病人感染的組織間隙不包含下列何者？(A)頰側間隙　(B)嚼肌間隙　(C)咽旁間隙　(D)頜下間隙

( )2. 請問病人接受的手術名稱為何？(A)腫瘤切除術　(B)齒切除術　(C)口內切開引流手術　(D)口外切開引流手術

( )3. 請問引起病人此次病症的主要原因？(A)蛀牙　(B)囊腫　(C)智齒周邊組織發炎　(D)牙周病

( )4. 請問病人所放置的引流管名稱為何？(A)CWV　(B)Penrose drain　(C)Foley drain　(D)Mini-hemovac

( )5. 請問病人後續需要接受的治療為何？(A)洗牙　(B)拔牙　(C)補牙　(D)根管治療

二、配合題

1. Osteomyelitis	(A)膿腫
2. Abscess	(B)智齒
3. Dental caries	(C)根管治療
4. Wisdom tooth	(D)腫脹
5. Gum	(E)張口困難
6. Scaling	(F)洗牙
7. Endodontic treatment	(G)骨髓炎
8. Flucuation	(H)蛀牙
9. Trismus	(I)波動感
10. Swelling	(J)牙齦

三、填充題

請寫出以下縮寫或生字之全文及中譯。

1. NPO _____

2. MMO _____

3. Offending tooth _____

4. I&D _____

5. POD _____

6. Lip numbness _____

7. IVF _____

8. Odontogenic _____

9. Parenteral antibiotics _____

10. Impacted tooth _____

學習評量解答
請掃描 QR Code

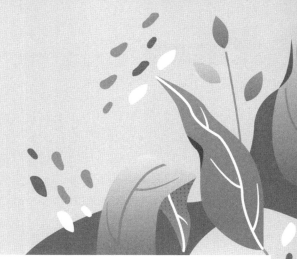

10 | CHAPTER

中醫病歷

作者 | 曹永昌、謝瓊慧

門診記錄

☑ 閱讀導引

1. 了解病人主訴與現在病史的關係。

2. 分析現在病史與過去病史之關聯性。

3. 分析現在病史、檢驗值與治療措施的合適性。

4. 能掌握閱讀會診單及照會回覆單之重點。

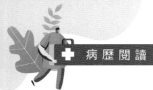
門診記錄

基本資料：

姓名：林〇〇　　　病歷號：300XXXXX　　　性別：男　　　年齡：63

婚姻：已婚　　　職業：公務員，已退休 3 年

家庭狀況：與太太同住，兒女皆已成家，偶幫忙照顧孫子。

身高：167 cm　　　體重：69 kg　　　初診日期：2023/06/11

主訴：

反覆胃脘悶痛，食物逆流，半夜胃抽筋已近半年。

現在病史：

63 歲男性有高尿酸血症已五年，每天服用西藥(Synorid (Allopurinol) 100 mg bid)控制，在 2022 年 6 月發現雙膝痛，西醫診斷為退化性關節炎，7 月時西醫開立 Brexin (Piroxicam)，病患斷斷續續服用了將近兩個月，之後出現胃悶痛、胃脹的症狀，但病患不以為意，只有停服 Brexin，無看醫師也無服用任何藥物緩解。

至 2023 年農曆年時胃部不舒服症狀明顯（胃悶痛、半夜胃絞痛、食物逆流），所以在 2/1 至三總檢查，胃鏡顯示：慢性胃炎、十二指腸炎、食道炎(GERD, LA grade B)。服用 Takepron (PPI)四個月後胃悶痛、食物逆流改善，但晚上仍會胃抽筋，之後醫師改開 Defense (Cimetidine) 300 mg bid，病患未服用，所以胃痛未再改善。

目前吃完食物後打嗝伴隨食物逆流，胃部悶脹不可坐。嚴重時整個食道都會有燒灼感伴隨胸悶、心下壓痛。吃多、坐下、前彎蹲下時症狀加重。半夜每 2 小時胃抽筋 1 次而醒來。

此外，病患聲音微沙啞且感覺鼻熱和咽喉熱。因上述困擾，故至本科就診。

過去病史：

心律不整史、高血壓（－）、糖尿病（－）、住院史（－）、手術史（－）。

檢查報告：

1. 2023/2/1 胃鏡：

   GERD, LA grade B, erosive gastritis, antrum esophagus mucosal breaks over EG junctuion ＞5 mm.

2. 2023/5/25 振興醫院冠狀動脈 CT: LAD calcified plaque & mixed plaque (proximal <30%，middle 30~50%)。

   →西醫給予 Licodin 100 mg (Ticlopidine)，但病患自行停服。

家族史：

1. 父母：無腸胃相關疾病。
2. 兄：糖尿病。

個人史：

1. 身高／體重：167 cm/69 kg、BMI：24.74、性情：易緊張、做事要求完美、睡眠：易入睡，但每兩小時胃抽筋醒來一次。
2. 睡眠時間：10:00 PM~5:00 AM。
3. 運動習慣：平日有運動習慣，走操場、爬山、騎腳踏車。
4. 飲食習慣：胃痛發作之前喝茶多，目前刺激性食物（包括茶）皆少吃，每餐 1~1.5 碗飯，飲食清淡。
5. 菸、酒、檳榔：（－）。

過敏史：

無食物、藥物過敏史。

中醫四診：

1. 望診：

   體型：微胖(167 cm/69 kg; BMI：24.74)、神態：精神可、面色：紅潤、眼睛：眼白色不黃，少血絲。下眼瞼色可。口唇：色正常、毛髮：白髮多，髮量少。四肢：無異常、舌質：舌紅、舌苔：苔黃膩。

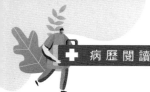

2. 聞診：

　　語音：聲微啞。氣味：無特殊異味。呼吸聲：無異常。

3. 問診：

(1) 情志：工作時壓力大、易緊張、做事要求完美，退休後壓力減輕，但還是會緊張、要求完美。

(2) 寒熱：怕熱，白天甚。

(3) 問汗：易流汗。40 多歲時心跳快(100+)，當時服用抑制交感神經藥物導致頭髮掉落。

(4) 頭身：頭暈（－），頭痛（－）。

(5) 耳目：近視 200 度，老花 200 度。耳鳴（－）。重聽（－）。

(6) 口咽：聲啞，喉嚨卡卡有痰，牙齒鬆動、易有酸感。

(7) 咽乾（－），口渴（－）。

(8) 胸腹：胸脇部易悶脹。

(9) 腰部：工作時因久坐腰部易痠。

(10) 睡眠：入睡可，多夢，每兩小時胃抽筋醒來一次。

(11) 二便：大便一日一行，需用力、不暢感、質硬，服軟便劑才可排淨。夜尿一次。

(12) 飲食：胃痛發作之前喝茶多，目前刺激性食物皆少吃，每餐 1~1.5 碗飯，飲食清淡。

4. 切診：

　　左脈：弦澀弱、右脈：弦澀弱。

整體回顧－時序圖

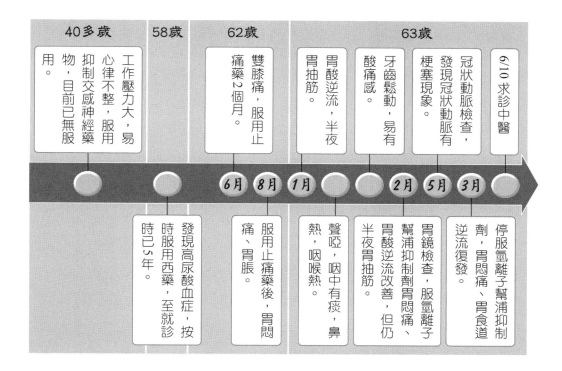

40多歲	58歲	62歲	63歲	

上方（時序軸上）：

40多歲
工作壓力大，易心律不整，服用抑制交感神經藥物，目前已無服用。

62歲（6月）
雙膝痛，服用止痛藥2個月。

62歲（1月）
胃酸逆流，半夜胃抽筋。

酸痛感。

牙齒鬆動，易有酸痛感。

63歲（5月）
發現冠狀動脈檢查，冠狀動脈有梗塞現象。

6/10 求診中醫

下方（時序軸下）：

58歲
發現高尿酸血症，按時服用西藥，至就診時已5年。

62歲（8月）
服用止痛藥後，胃悶痛、胃脹。

聲啞，咽中有痰，鼻熱，咽喉熱。

半夜胃抽筋。

63歲（2月）
胃鏡檢查，服氫離子幫浦抑制劑胃悶痛、胃酸逆流改善，但仍

63歲（3月）
停服氫離子幫浦抑制劑，胃悶痛、胃食道逆流復發。

整體回顧-LQQOPERA：

L： 發作部位在胃、食道。

Q： 幾乎持續發作。食後和半夜時較嚴重。

Q： 食後易打嗝、食物逆流、胃部悶脹不可坐。半夜每兩小時胃絞痛一次。

O： 慢性，反覆發作。

P： 2022 年服用止痛藥兩個月後發生，易緊張、要求完美。

E： 吃多、坐下、前彎蹲下時加重。

R： 服用氫離子幫浦抑制劑緩解。

A： 伴隨聲啞，喉嚨有梗塞感，喉熱，鼻熱，胸**脇**悶脹，牙齒鬆動、易酸痛。

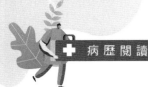
整體回顧：

1. 當吃多時，情況會更加嚴重，嚴重時整個食道都會有燒灼感伴隨胸悶、心下壓痛。

2. 胃痛發作之前喝茶多，目前刺激性食物皆少吃（包括茶），每餐 1~1.5 碗飯，飲食清淡。

3. 個性易緊張，做事要求完美。

4. 怕熱，白天甚。易流汗。

5. 大便一日一行，需用力、不暢感、質硬，需用軟便劑。

6. 舌質：舌紅。舌苔：苔黃膩。

7. 脈：弦澀弱。

診斷：

1. 西醫：530.81－胃食道逆流。

2. 中醫：辨病－胃脘痛、吞酸。辨證－肝（膽）胃不和，痰熱上逆。

3. 治則：疏肝和胃，清熱滌痰。

病機四大要素分析：

1. 理－病因：
   (1) 內因（內傷七情）：個性易緊張，要求完美，之前工作壓力大。
   (2) 不內外因（飲食失調）：喜飲茶。服用止痛藥過多，傷害胃黏膜。

2. 理－病位：
   (1) 臟腑：肝（膽）、胃。
   (2) 解剖：胃、食道、十二指腸。

3. 理－病性：
   (1) 主證：食後打嗝伴隨食物逆流，嚴重時食道有燒灼感，半夜每 2 小時胃抽筋 1 次而醒來。舌紅，苔黃膩。脈弦澀弱。
   (2) 次證：胸脇悶、心下壓痛。聲音沙啞且感覺鼻熱和咽喉熱。咽中梗痰。牙齒鬆動、易感覺酸痛感。

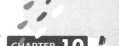

4. 理－病勢：
(1) 平時易緊張，要求完美，導致肝失條達，膽失疏泄，氣鬱化火，故致畏熱、多汗、大便硬而不暢及心跳過快史。
(2) 喜飲茶，飲食失節，加上服用止痛藥過度，造成脾胃損傷，濕熱內蘊。熱灼成痰，故致胃酸過多，鼻熱、咽喉熱，咽喉有痰梗塞、聲啞，舌質紅，苔黃膩。
(3) 痰熱上擾於心，故多夢。
(4) 肝膽氣機不暢，阻於經脈，故致胸悶、胸脅部悶脹、脈帶弦象；氣滯不行，久而血瘀，導致冠動阻塞，故而脈澀弱。
(5) 肝膽之氣橫逆犯胃，故致胃失和降，胃氣上逆，造成食後打嗝、食物逆流及食道燒灼感等症。
　　肝主筋，肝氣阻滯，不能「淫氣於筋」，加之胃熱灼傷筋脈，故致夜間胃脘痙攣。

病因病機圖

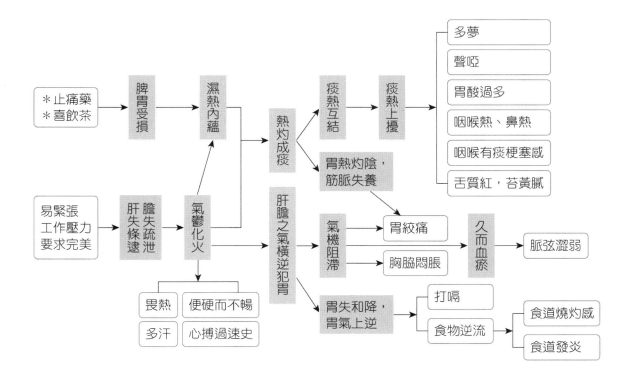

法：

疏肝和胃，清熱滌痰。

方藥：

溫肝湯 6g，芍藥甘草湯 6g，黃連 2g，牡蠣 1.5g，香附 1.5g，一天三次，共服七天。

護理小幫手

Little Helper

溫膽湯

【組成】半夏 10 克、橘紅 15 克、茯苓 8 克、甘草 5 克、竹茹 10 克、枳實 10 克、生薑 10 克、大棗 2 枚。

【功用】行氣化痰，調和膽胃。

【主治】膽胃不和、痰濁內擾證。虛煩失眠、胸悶有痰，噁心嘔吐、呃逆、或驚悸不寧、口苦、苔膩、脈弦滑。

芍藥甘草湯

【組成】白芍藥 4 兩甘草炙 4 兩

【功用】柔肝益陰、緩急止痛。

【主治】1.肝陰不足、剋犯脾土、腹拘急而痛。2.陰液不足、筋脈失養、手足攣急。

黃連

【性味、歸經】苦，寒。歸心、肝、胃、大腸經。

【功效】清熱燥濕，瀉火解毒。

【主治】

1. 本品大苦大寒，清熱燥濕之力勝于黃芩，尤長於清中焦濕火鬱結，善除脾胃大腸濕熱，為治濕熱瀉痢要藥。
2. 用於熱盛火熾、高熱煩躁。本品瀉火解毒，尤善清心經實火。
3. 本品善清胃火，可用於胃火熾盛的嘔吐。

【現代藥理】本品含小檗鹼（黃連素）、甲基黃連鹼等多種生物鹼。黃連有很廣的抗菌範圍，其中對痢疾桿菌的抑制作用最強。並能增強白細胞的吞噬能力，又有降壓、利膽、解熱、鎮靜、鎮痛、抗利尿、局部麻痺等作用。此外，對血管平滑肌有鬆弛作用，對子宮、膀胱、腸胃道平滑肌鬆弛呈興奮作用。

牡蠣

【性味、歸經】鹹、澀、微寒。歸肝、腎經。

【功效】平肝潛陽，軟堅散結，收斂固澀。

【主治】

1. 用於肝陽上亢，頭暈目眩。本品鹹寒質重，似石決明之平肝潛陽作用。

2. 牡蠣味鹹，軟堅散結。用於痰核，瘰癧，癥瘕積聚等證。

3. 用於滑脫諸證。本品味澀，煅用有與煅龍骨相仿的收斂固澀作用。

4. 煅牡蠣有收斂制酸作用，可治胃痛泛酸，以之與烏賊骨、浙貝母共為細末，內服取效。

【現代藥理】本品含 80~95%的碳酸鈣、磷酸鈣及硫酸鈣，并含鎂、鋁、硅、氧化鐵及有機質等。煅燒後碳酸鹽分解，產生氧化鈣等，有機質則被破壞。所含鈣鹽有抗酸及輕度鎮靜、消炎作用。對胃及十二指腸潰瘍有一定療效。尚可增強免疫力。

香附

【性味、歸經】辛、微苦、微甘、平。歸肝、脾、三焦經。

【功效】疏肝理氣，調經止痛。

【主治】

1. 用於氣滯脅痛，腹痛。本品辛能通行、苦能疏泄、微甘緩急，為疏肝解鬱、行氣止痛之要藥。

2. 用於肝鬱月經不調，痛經，乳房脹痛。本品有疏肝解鬱、行氣散結、調經止痛之功。

【現代藥理】

1. 本品含揮發油。此外尚含生物鹼、黃酮類及三萜類等。

2. 其水煎劑有降低腸管緊張性和拮抗乙醯膽鹼的作用。

3. 香附油對金黃色葡萄球菌有抑制作用。其提取物對某些真菌有抑制作用。

4. 其總生物鹼、甙類、黃酮類及酚類化合物的水溶液有強心及降低血壓的作用。

衛教：

1. 調整生活方式

　(1) 飲食習慣：避免食用下列食品：

　　．柳橙汁、葡萄柚汁和番茄汁。

　　．油炸或高脂肪食品。

- 辛辣食物。
- 酒、菸、碳酸飲料及咖啡。
- 過甜之食品如巧克力。

(2) 生活型態調整：

- 維持適當體重及適當的飲食習慣。
- 戒菸。
- 不穿太緊身的食物或束繫皮帶。
- 避免彎腰提重物。
- 避免在睡前 1~2 小時內進食。
- 躺臥時，頭部宜墊高 15~20 公分左右。

治療過程：

6/11、6/18、7/2、7/16、7/30、8/27、10/8、11/12、12/19、1/21、2/18 共 11 次。

6/11（初診）	6/18
・S：食後胃脹、打嗝、逆流，食道灼熱感，伴隨胸悶，食多症狀加重。鼻熱、咽喉熱、咽中有痰、聲微啞。平素易緊張。半夜每兩小時胃絞痛而醒來，多夢。大便一日一行，不暢偏硬，需使用軟便劑。 ・O：舌紅，苔黃膩。 　　脈弦澀弱	・S：反胃(-)，半夜已無胃抽筋，可一覺到天亮，多夢改善。呼氣時鼻腔熱，音啞。大便平。 ・O：舌淡紅，苔黃膩。 　　脈弦。
A：疏肝和胃、清熱滌痰 P：溫膽湯　　　　6g 　　芍藥甘草湯　　6g 　　黃連　　　　　2g　─ 3×7天 　　牡蠣　　　　　1.5g 　　香附　　　　　1.5g	A：疏肝和胃、清熱滌痰 P：溫膽湯　　　　7.5g 　　芍藥甘草湯　　7.5g 　　黃連　　　　　2.5g　─ 4×14天 　　牡蠣　　　　　1.5g 　　香附　　　　　1.5g

7/2

7/2
- S：食後逆流已大減，食道灼熱感減。呼氣仍鼻熱。半夜胃絞痛已無，多夢減。大便平，不需使用軟便劑。反胃(−)，噯氣(−)，泛酸(−)。5/25冠狀動脈檢查顯示輕微阻塞，但未服用西醫開的抗凝血劑。
- O：舌淡紅，苔薄黃，裂紋。
  左脈弦，右脈弦澀弱

7/16
- S：食後逆流已大減，但食冰或甜則聲啞明顯。鼻熱和咽喉熱仍有。胃抽筋未再犯。
- O：舌淡紅，苔黃膩。
  脈弦細澀弱。

7/16

A：疏肝和胃、清熱滌痰、活血化瘀
P：溫膽湯　　　　　6g ⎤
　　芍藥甘草湯　　　6g ⎥
　　黃連　　　　　　2g ⎥
　　牡蠣　　　　　1.5g ⎥ 4×14天
　　香附　　　　　1.5g ⎥
　　白芨　　　　　1.5g ⎥
　　丹參　　　　　1.5g ⎥
　　三七　　　　　　3g ⎦

7/30

- S：食後逆流已減，食道灼熱感減。但早上空腹喝水好發胃灼熱。鼻熱、咽喉熱稍減。咽中有痰、鼻微啞仍有。半夜胃絞痛已無，大便平。眠可。
- O：舌淡紅，苔薄白，裂紋。
  脈弦澀

A：疏肝和胃、清熱滌痰、活血化瘀
P：溫膽湯　　　　　6g ⎤
　　芍藥甘草湯　　　5g ⎥
　　黃連　　　　　　2g ⎥
　　牡蠣　　　　　　2g ⎥ 4×28天
　　香附　　　　　1.5g ⎥
　　白芨　　　　　1.5g ⎥
　　丹參　　　　　1.5g ⎥
　　三七　　　　　　3g ⎦

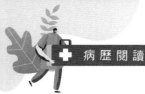

病 歷 閱 讀　Understanding Medical Records

8/27	10/8	11/12

8/27
- S：胃中偶有熱氣。七夕吃麻油雞酒後逆流、胃痛發生一次。聲啞減。鼻熱和咽喉熱減。腹脹(–)，絞痛(–)，二便平，眠可。家中測量　BP:115~120/75，PR:65~69。
- O：舌淡紅，苔薄白，中後段黃膩。脈弦

10/8
- S：胃熱改善，但食月餅泛酸，胃痛無，食冰或甜則聲啞。鼻熱和咽喉熱減。
- O：舌淡紅，苔薄白，中裂。脈弦

11/12
- S：胃熱已無。但飲一次咖啡又犯胃熱、音啞及咽熱一次。泛酸(–)，鼻熱(–)。二便平，眠可。
- O：舌淡紅，苔薄白，裂紋。脈弦

A：疏肝和胃、清熱滌痰、活血化瘀
P：溫膽湯　　　　6g
　　芍藥甘草湯　4.5g
　　黃連　　　　2.5g
　　牡蠣　　　　2g
　　香附　　　　1.5g ├ 4×28天
　　白芨　　　　1.5g
　　丹參　　　　1.5g
　　三七　　　　3g

12/19

- S：夜間胃抽筋本已無，前幾日吃乳酪蛋糕後半夜發生一次，但瞬間緩解。吃太飽胃脹痛，起立走動半小時緩解。飲咖啡或食乳酪蛋糕後仍易咽熱。泛酸(–)，胃灼熱(–)。二便平，眠可。
- O：舌質淡紅，舌苔前段薄黃，中後段薄黃膩、中有裂紋。脈弦無力

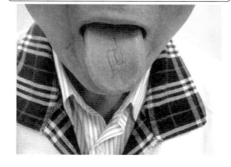

A：疏肝和胃、清熱滌痰、活血化瘀
P：溫膽湯　　　　6g
　　芍藥甘草湯　4.5g
　　黃連　　　　2.5g
　　牡蠣　　　　2g
　　香附　　　　1.5g ├ 4×28天
　　白芨　　　　1.5g
　　丹參　　　　1.5g
　　三七　　　　3g

1/21	2/18

1/21
- S：1/9植牙，服3天抗生素後胃痛，停藥後又緩解。飢餓時胃脘不適，腹脹(−)，泛酸(−)，半夜胃抽筋(−)，食甜泛酸逆流感和胃脘痛已不會發作。餐後腹脹已無。大便平。
  家中測量BP:110~120/75~80。
- O：舌淡紅，苔薄白，裂紋。
  脈弦澀

2/18
- S：胃痛未犯，但飢餓時胃脘不適發作1~2次，服中藥後立刻緩解。晨起口苦。腹脹(−)，食甜泛酸(−)，半夜胃抽筋。二便平。
- O：舌淡紅，苔薄白，裂紋。
  脈弦

A：疏肝和胃、清熱滌痰、活血化瘀
P：
溫膽湯	6g
芍藥甘草湯	4.5g
黃連	2.5g
牡蠣	2g
香附	1.5g
白芨	1.5g
丹參	1.5g
三七	3g

4×28天

註：本文感謝吳宛容醫師整理。

219

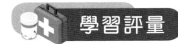

一、選擇題

( )1. 有關林先生到門診時現病史中之敘述，何者為非？(A)高尿酸血症已七年 (B)西醫診斷退化性關節炎　(C)胃鏡顯示：慢性胃炎、十二指腸炎、食道炎 (D)半夜每 2 小時胃抽筋 1 次

( )2. 門診醫師對於林先生望診觀察，何者為是？(A)眼睛：眼白色不黃，少血絲 (B)舌質：舌紅　(C)舌苔：苔黃膩　(D)以上皆是

( )3. 門診醫師對於林先生聞診觀察，何者為是？(A)語音：聲微啞　(B)氣味：無 特殊異味　(C)呼吸聲：無異常　(D)以上皆是

( )4. 門診醫師對於林先生問診情形，何者為非？(A)胸脇部易悶脹　(B)少汗 (C)大便一日一行　(D)胃痛發作之前喝茶多

( )5. 門診醫師對於林先生切診情形，何者為是？(A)左脈：弦澀弱　(B)右脈：弦 澀弱　(C)以上皆是

( )6. 溫膽湯主治何者為非？(A)膽胃不和、痰濁內擾證　(B)虛煩失眠　(C)氣滯 脅痛，腹痛　(D)驚悸不寧

( )7. 黃連主治何者為是？(A)治濕熱瀉痢　(B)瀉火毒　(C)善清胃火　(D)以上皆 是

( )8. 牡蠣主治何者為是？(A)用於肝陽上亢，頭暈目眩　(B)用於滑脫諸證　(C) 用於痰核，瘰癧等證　(D)以上皆是

( )9. 對於林先生衛教何者為非？(A)避免在睡前 1~2 小時內進食　(B)躺臥時頭部 宜墊高 15~20 公分左右　(C)不穿太緊身的食物或束繫皮帶　(D)宜吃辛辣食 物

學習評量解答
請掃描 QR Code

11 | CHAPTER

門診病歷

作者｜梁繼權、郭彥志、謝如蘭

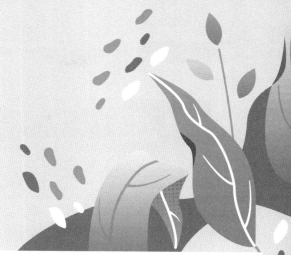

☑ 閱讀導引

1. 了解門診病歷的書寫原則。
2. 了解初診記錄與複診記錄的差異。
3. 了解各科病歷的記錄重點。
4. 了解各科疾病的治療方法。

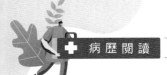

11-1 Neurology

Initial Visit

2023-2-5   2:40 p.m.

Chief Complaint:

Sudden onset left side weakness in this morning.

Present Illness:

This 45 year-old man has history of **mitral valve insufficiency** and **paroxysmal atrial fibrillation**, and had received anticoagulant treatment since 7 years ago. In order to get promotion, he worked very hard. However, it made him forget to take his medication several times a month. This morning, he experienced right side weakness and difficulty to speak clearly, while those symptoms disappeared two hours later. Since his father died of a **stroke**, his wife really worry about his condition.

Past History:

1. **RHD** with **MR**, **AF**(+).

2. Hospitalization: Denied.

3. Operation: Denied.

Personal History:

1. Medication: Coumadin® (Warfarin) 2.5 mg/tab 2# QD PO.

2. Alcohol (seldom), smoking (-), betel nut (-).

3. Allergic history: No known drug or food allergy.

Family History:

1. Father: Hypertension, died of hemorrhagic stroke at age of 65 years old.

2. Mother: Hypertension, died of cervical cancer.

3. Sibling: 4, elder brother has hypertension and one episode of **TIA**.

Review of System:

Left side weakness, **dysarthria**, no urine or stool incontinence.

Physical Examination:

1. General appearance: Anxious. BP: 160/110 mmHg, PR: 80/min.

2. HEENT: Non-anemic conjunctiva; anicteric sclera; papillary light reflex: prompt in both eyes.

3. Neck: Supple, no jugular vein engorgement; no palpable lymph node; normal sized thyroid gland; no carotid bruit.

4. Chest: Symmetric expansion; clear breath sounds.

5. Heart: Irregular heart beats; **gr.** 3/6 **systolic blowing murmur** at apex, left sternal border, axilla and upper back.

6. Abdomen: Flat; normoactive bowel sound; no tenderness or rebound tenderness; no **hepatosplenomegaly**.

7. Extremities: No deformity, no edema, free joint movement.

8. Peripheral pulsations: Normal and equal in carotid, brachial, popliteal and dorsalis pedis arteries.

9. Neurological examination: Normal muscle power, no sensory loss or dysesthesia, cranial nerves no abnormal finding.

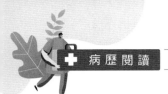

Impression:

1. Stroke (transit ischemic attack).

2. Rheumatic heart disease with mitral valve insufficiency and paroxysmal atrial fibrillation.

Management:

1. Educate the importance of drug compliance.

2. Check prothrombin time and International Normalized Ratio (INR).

3. Risk factor evaluation (monitor blood pressure, check serum lipid profile and blood sugar).

4. Arrange carotid duplex examination.

5. OPD follow-up.

Attending Physician: ×××

關鍵字彙 Keywords

字　彙	原　文	中　譯
Mitral valve insufficiency		僧帽瓣閉鎖不全
Paroxysmal atrial fibrillation		陣發性心房纖維顫動
Stroke		中風
RHD	rheumatic heart disease	風濕性心臟病
MR	mitral regurgitation	二尖瓣逆流
AF	atrial fibrillation.	心房纖維顫動
TIA	transit ischemic attack	暫時性腦缺氧
Dysarthria		構音困難
gr.	grade	分級
Systolic blowing murmur		收縮期心雜音
Hepatosplenomegaly	hepat，肝 splen，脾 megaly，腫	肝脾腫大

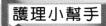

護理小幫手　　　　　　　　　　　　　　　　　　　　　　Little Helper

認識腦中風

　　腦部的血液循環主要經由頸部的內頸動脈與脊椎動脈所供應。中風可分為兩大類：栓塞性和出血性。栓塞是由於血液供應中斷，而腦出血是由於腦血管破裂或不正常的血管結構。80%的中風是由於腦栓塞，其餘的是由於出血所致。中風的危險因素包括高齡、高血壓、前中風史或暫時性腦缺氧 (TIA)、糖尿病、高膽固醇、吸菸、心房纖維顫動。

　　如果懷疑中風，可以評估看看臉部是否有任何下垂或肌肉張力喪失；要求病人閉眼，伸直手臂 30 秒－如果病人中風，您可能會看到一隻手臂緩慢下移；聽病人講話是否含糊等方式來初步測驗。進一步的診斷則需要藉由 CT 或 MRI 等影像檢查來協助確立診斷。

　　本個案發生腦中風的危險因子包括高血壓、高脂血症、心房纖維顫動。有心房纖維顫動的病人突發中風，應考慮左心房栓子所引發的中風，並以抗凝血劑(Warfarin)治療，防止心房栓子形成。

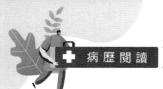

Follow-Up Visit

2023-2-7　　9:34 a.m.

Chief Complaint and Problems:

For result and follow-up.

Physical Examination:

1. BP: 150/96 mmHg, PR: 90/min, irregular.

2. No carotid bruits, heart murmur: No change.

3. Normal muscle power, no hypoesthesia or dysesthesia.

Laboratory data:

1. Coagulation

Date	Prothrombin time	INR
2023-2-6	15 sec	1.5

2. BCS

Date	Total cholesterol	Triglyceride	LDL-C	blood suger AC
2023-2-6	258 mg/dL	315 mg/dL	160 mg/dL	98 mg/dL

3. Carotid duplex: >50% stenosis at right common carotid artery.

Diagnosis:

1. Stroke (transit ischemic attack).

2. Rheumatic heart disease with mitral valve insufficiency and paroxysmal atrial fibrillation.

3. Hypertension.

4. Hyperlipidemia.

5. Right carotid stenosis.

Management:

1. Remind regular warfarin usage and monitor INR.

2. Valsartan 80 mg/tab 1# QD PO.

3. Atrovastatin 10 mg/tab 1# QD PO.

4. Diet control.

Attending Physician: ✕ ✕ ✕

學習評量

一、選擇題

(　)1. 下列何者並非本個案發生腦中風的可改變危險因子？(A)hypertension (B)hyperlipidemia　(C)atrial fibrillation　(D)age

(　)2. 下列何者並非本個案病史？(A)RHD　(B)COPD　(C)AF　(D)MR

(　)3. 下列何者並非個案出現 TIA 的徵候？(A)left side weakness　(B)dysarthria (C)symptoms disappeared after two hours　(D)dysesthesia

(　)4. 請問此個案的心雜音為第幾級？(A)1　(B)2　(C)3　(D)4

(　)5. 請問此個案的總頸動脈超音波結果為何？(A)狹窄＞50%　(B)狹窄＞30% (C)狹窄＞20%　(D)normal

二、填充題

請寫出以下縮寫或生字之全文及中譯。

1. Mitral valve insufficiency_____

2. Paroxysmal atrial fibrillation_____

3. Stroke_____

4. Dysarthria_____

5. Systolic blowing murmur_____

6. Hepatosplenomegaly_____

7. RHD_____

8. MR_____

9. AF_____

10. TIA_____

學習評量解答
請掃描 QR Code

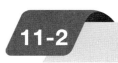 **Chest Medicine**

Initial Visit

2023-3-15   11:40 a.m.

Chief Complaint:

Cough and dyspnea for about one week.

Present Illness:

This 54 year-old housewife has developed **nonproductive cough** since one week ago. She has also experienced general malaise, poor appetite and exertional dyspea. At first, she thought that she just had a common cold and took some **over-the-counter cold medication** for relief. However, dyspnea became more prominent in the recent two days, and she was unable to tolerate her usual works such as sweeping the floor or carrying groceries from the market. There was no fever nor chills in this episode. She had an operation for pulmonary tuberculosis many years ago, and high blood pressure discovered by a health check, but hasn't received any medical treatment yet.

Past History:

1. High blood pressure without medical control.
2. Hospitalization and operation for **pulmonary TB** 10 years ago.

Personal History:

1. Denied any long-term medication, alcohol consumption, smoking and betel nut chewing.
2. No drug or food allergy history.

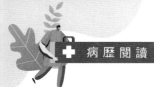
Family History:

Father and mother had pulmonary TB. Father died of massive bleeding due to **hemoptysis** 15 years ago.

Review of System:

Nonproductive cough(+), general malaise(+), poor appetite(+), exertional dyspnea(+).

Physical Examination:

1. BP: 180/118 mmHg, BT: 37.1℃, PR: 96/min, RR: 20/min.
2. HEENT: Conjunctiva: not anemic; sclera: anicteric.
3. Neck: Supple. No jugular vein engorgement; no palpable lymph node; normal sized thyroid gland. No carotid bruit.
4. Chest: Symmetric expansion. Dullness on percussion over lower lungs. Breath sound: Decreased in both lower lung fields, crackles was heard in the left lung.
5. Heart: Regular heart beats; no murmur; normal S_1 and S_2, no S_3 or S_4.
6. Abdomen: Globular; normoactive bowel sound; shifting dullness(+); no tenderness or rebound tenderness; no hepatosplenomegaly.
7. Extremities: No deformity or limitation of joint movement. Bilateral lower limb pitting edema(+).

Impression:

1. Suspected pulmonary consolidation or pleural effusion.
2. Suspected **CHF**.

Management:

1. CXR PA.

2. Check CBC, WBC differential count and BCS including creatinine, blood urea nitrogen, potassium, sodium, ALT, AST and albumin.

3. Enalapril 10 mg/tab 1# QD PO for 3 day.

4. Furosemide 40 mg/tab 1# QD PO for 3 day.

5. Make appointment 3 days later.

Attending Physician: ×××

關鍵字彙 Keywords

字　彙	原　文	中　譯
Nonproductive cough		乾咳
Over-the-counter cold medication		感冒成藥
Pulmonary TB	pulmonary tuberculosis	肺結核
Hemoptysis	hemo-，血	咳血
CHF	congestive heart failure	充血性心衰竭
Tachycardia	tachy-，快 -cardia，心	心搏過快
Lobectomy	-ectomy，切除術	肺葉切除術

護理小幫手

Little Helper

認識肋膜積水

　　肋膜積水是液體蓄積在壁層肋膜與臟層肋膜之間形成的肋膜腔中，由液體形成機轉與液體之成分組成可分為漏出液與滲出液兩大類。滲出液性質的肋膜積水與肺炎、肺動脈栓塞、尿毒症等有關；漏出液性質的肋膜積水與肝硬化、腎病症候群、低蛋白血症等有關。臨床會出現聽診時呼吸音減少或消失，叩診出現濁音(dullness)，CXR 顯示肋骨和橫膈間角度(costophrenic angle)變鈍等症狀。

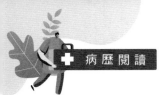
Follow-Up Visit

2023-3-18　　9:30 a.m.

Chief Complaint and Problems:

1. Dyspnea progressed.
2. Unable to lie down to sleep due to dyspnea.

Physical Examination:

1. BP: 160/110 mmHg，PR: 120/min, RR: 30/min.
2. Chest: Accessory muscle breathing, decreased breath sounds at bilateral middle and lower lungs.
3. Heart: **Tachycardia**, no audible heart murmur.
4. Abdomen: More protruded, shifting dullness(+).
5. Lower extremities: Pitting edema at bilateral ankles and lower legs(+).

Laboratory Data:

1. CXR: Opacification of bilateral lower lungs suspected bilateral pleural effusion, suspected right upper lung **lobectomy**, borderline heart size.
2. CBC

Date	RBC	WBC	Hb	Platelet	MCV	HCT	MCHC	MCH
2023-3-15	4.05 M/uL	12,500/uL	11.5 g/dL	565,000/uL	84.5 fL	43.5%	30.5 g/dL	25.6 pg

3. Differential Count

Date	Neutrophil	Lymphocyte	Monocyte	Eosinophil	Basophil
2023-3-15	85.5%	10.5%	2.6%	1.2%	0.2%

4. BCS

Date	Creatinine	BUN	ALT	AST	Sodium	Potassium	Albumin
2023-3-15	1.3 mg/L	25.4 mg/dL	76 U/L	65 U/L	145 mEq/L	4.5 mEq/L	3.8 g/dL

Diagnosis:

1. Bilateral pleural effusion, cause to be determined.
2. Suspected impending respiratory failure.

Management:

1. Oxygen supply with O_2 mask 10 L/min.
2. Transfer to emergency department immediately.

Attending Physician: × × ×

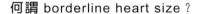

護理小幫手　　　　　　　　　　　　　　　　　　Little Helper

何謂 borderline heart size？

　　當胸部 X 光判讀出現 borderline heart size（邊緣性心臟大小），意思是指心臟的大小在正常的上限，意味著實際的心臟大小可能正常或略有增加。一般胸部 X 光片評估心臟是否擴大是以心臟大小是否比胸腔大二分之一，borderline heart size 即表示心臟大約是胸腔的一半，若欲進一步了解心臟實際是否有擴大的現象，需進一步做其他詳細檢查。

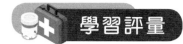

學習評量

一、選擇題

(　)1. 下列何者為個案入院的主訴？(A)cough and dyspnea for about one month (B)good appetite　(C)fever and chill　(D)exertional dyspea

(　)2. 下列何者並非此個案肋膜積水的症狀？(A)resonance on percussion over lower lungs　(B)breath sound decreased　(C)crackles in the left lung (D)exertional dyspnea

(　)3. 下列何者並非此個案的個人與家族史？(A)pulmonary TB　(B)high blood pressure with medical control　(C)no drug or food allergy history　(D)father and mother had pulmonary TB

(　)4. 下列何者為此個案於三天後複診時的病情變化？(A)normal breath sounds (B)dyspnea progressed　(C)murmur　(D)regular heart beats

(　)5. 下列何者為個案於複診時醫師的處置？(A)oxygen　30L/min　(B)take medicine　(C)transfer to ER　(D)follow-up 3 days later

二、填充題

請寫出以下縮寫或生字之全文及中譯。

1. Exertional dyspea＿＿＿＿＿＿＿＿＿＿＿＿＿＿＿＿＿＿＿＿＿

2. Hemoptysis＿＿＿＿＿＿＿＿＿＿＿＿＿＿＿＿＿＿＿＿＿＿＿＿

3. Pleural effusion＿＿＿＿＿＿＿＿＿＿＿＿＿＿＿＿＿＿＿＿＿

4. Tachycardia＿＿＿＿＿＿＿＿＿＿＿＿＿＿＿＿＿＿＿＿＿＿＿

5. Lobectomy＿＿＿＿＿＿＿＿＿＿＿＿＿＿＿＿＿＿＿＿＿＿＿＿

6. Respiratory failure＿＿＿＿＿＿＿＿＿＿＿＿＿＿＿＿＿＿＿＿

7. TB＿＿＿＿＿＿＿＿＿＿＿＿＿＿＿＿＿＿＿＿＿＿＿＿＿＿＿

8. CHF＿＿＿＿＿＿＿＿＿＿＿＿＿＿＿＿＿＿＿＿＿＿＿＿＿＿＿

學習評量解答
請掃描 QR Code

11-3 　 Cardiovascular Medicine

Initial Visit

2023-3-1 　 9:45 a.m.

Chief Complaint:

Chest pain for about two months.

Present Illness:

This 65 year-old man has experienced intermittent compression pain at his left chest for about two months. Usually, the pain occurs during exertion such as climbing stairs or jogging, and disappears 2~5 minutes later when he takes a rest. Sometimes it would radiate to his jaw and neck. He didn't have any cough or dyspnea, and denied other major system disease except hypertension and hyperlipidemia which were diagnosed a few years ago without regular treatment. During this month, he felt his exercising endurance has decreased. Therefore, he came to our clinic for help.

Past History:

1. Hypertension (BP about 160/100 mmHg), hyperlipidemia (total cholesterol around 250 mg/dL).
2. Denied history of hospitalization and major operation.

Personal History:

1. Medication: Denied.
2. Alcohol: 100 mL red wine/day for more than 20 years, smoking: 0.5 PPD for 15 years, but quit 20 years ago, betel nut(-).
3. Allergic history: Only to seafood (skin rash).

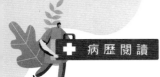

Family History:

1. Father: Died of coronary artery disease at age of 60.

2. Mother: No systemic disease; now is 90 years old.

3. Siblings: Non-contributory.

Review of System:

Left chest pain, compressive in nature, aggravated by exertion and alleviated by rest.

Physical Examination:

1. BP: 160/96 mmHg, PR: 80/min.

2. Conjunctiva: Not anemic, no carotid bruits, no goiter.

3. Chest: Normal breath sounds, no crackle or wheezing.

4. Heart: Regular heart beats, no murmur.

5. Abdomen: No hepatosplenomegaly.

6. Extremities: No pitting edema.

7. Peripheral pulsations: Normal and equal.

Impression:

1. Chest pain, suspected ischemic heart disease.

2. Hypertension and hyperlipidemia.

Management:

1. Monitor blood pressure at home.

2. Check serum lipid profile, serum creatinine, ALT, and blood sugar.

3. Arrange EKG and treadmill exercise test.

4. Low salt and cholesterol diet.

Attending Physician: <u>××× </u>

護理小幫手　　　　　　　　　　　　　　　　　　　　Little Helper

認識缺血性心臟病

　　心臟供血不足而引起的疾病稱為缺血性心臟病。冠狀動脈是主要供應心臟血液與養分的血管，冠狀動脈內壁上產生粥樣硬化斑塊，而使這些動脈受到阻塞所致時，即會引起心臟缺血，又稱冠狀動脈心臟病。引起冠狀動脈硬化的因素有：膽固醇過高、吸菸、高血壓、糖尿病、精神壓抑、肥胖等。心肌梗塞即是當冠狀動脈粥樣硬化時造成心絞痛(angina pectoris)或部分的心肌壞死。典型心絞痛疼痛的位置通常位於胸部的中間，疼痛的性質為緊縮、陣陣刺痛，而且疼痛會放射到其他的部位，如左臂、左頸，且疼痛持續的時間通常都為 2~3 分鐘，很少超過 10 分鐘。

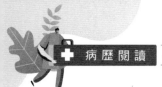
Follow-Up Visit

2023-3-8　　11:30 a.m.

Chief Complaint and Problems:

For result and follow-up.

Physical Examination:

1. BP: 158/96 mmHg, PR: 80/min regular.

2. No other positive physical finding.

Laboratory Data:

1. BCS

Date	Total cholesterol	Triglyceride	HDL-C	Glucose AC	Creatinine	ALT
2023-3-2	315 mg/dL	140 mg/dL	35 mg/dL	80 mg/dL	0.8 mg/L	41U/L

2. EKG: Sinus rhythm, 85 beats/min, non-specific ST-T change.

3. Treadmill exercise test: Significant ST depression at V1 to V3 in second stage of exercise.

Diagnosis:

1. Ischemic heart disease.

2. Hypertension.

3. Hyperlipidemia.

Management:

1. Arrange admission for coronary catheterization.

2. Aspirin 100 mg/tab 1# QD PO.

3. Nadolol 40 mg/tab 1# QD PO.

4. Atrovastatin 20 mg/tab 1# QD PO.

Attending Physician: ×××

 護理小幫手

Little Helper

缺血性心臟病的診斷與治療

　　缺血性心臟病的診斷除了依臨床症狀外，還可利用運動踏板心電圖 (treadmill exercise test)、心臟超音波或核子醫學心臟灌注的檢查來輔助診斷，心導管檢查(coronary catheterization)是目前診斷冠狀動脈疾病最準確的方法。運動踏板心電圖是以運動方式使心臟需氧量增加，此時心肌可能因缺氧而導致心絞痛，心肌缺氧的異常狀況會顯示在心電圖上，故嚴重心律不整患者不宜進行。心導管檢查除了可用於診斷疾病外，亦可評估冠狀動脈的狹窄程度、擴張狹窄的動脈、放置冠狀動脈支架作為治療的方式。

　　治療心絞痛的方法有藥物治療和手術治療。缺血性心臟病病人高血壓治療的首選藥物為 β-受體阻斷劑，如果病人血管狹窄的嚴重程度小於 70%，則藥物治療即可，血管狹窄嚴重可施行冠狀動脈繞道手術(CABG)。

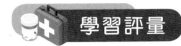

學習評量

一、選擇題

( )1. 下列缺血性心臟病症狀中，何者並非此個案的症狀？(A)intermittent compression pain　(B)the pain usually occurs during exertion　(C)pain would disappear 30 minutes later when he took a rest　(D)the pain would radiate to his jaw and neck

( )2. 下列何者並非此個案的缺血性心臟病危險因素？(A)hypertension　(B)DM (C)hyperlipidemia　(D)smoking

( )3. 下列何者並非缺血性心臟病的診斷依據？(A)EKG　(B)catheterization (C)treadmill exercise test　(D)CXR

( )4. 缺血性心臟病病人高血壓治療的首選藥物為何？(A)β-受體阻斷劑　(B)α-受體阻斷劑　(C)利尿劑　(D)阿斯匹靈

( )5. 下列何者飲食較適合此個案？(A)low salt and cholesterol diet　(B)DM diet (C)element diet　(D)liquid diet

二、填充題

請寫出以下縮寫或生字之全文及中譯。

1. Hypertension_____

2. Hyperlipidemia_____

3. Cholesterol_____

4. Coronary artery disease_____

5. Ischemic heart disease_____

6. Treadmill exercise test_____

7. Angina_____

8. Coronary catheterization_____

學習評量解答
請掃描 QR Code

11-4 Nephrology

Initial Visit

2023-2-5   10:00 a.m.

Chief Complaint:

Numbness of feet and swelling of ankles since yesterday morning.

Present Illness:

This 60 year-old man has history of **DM** for more than 15 years. About seven days ago, he had suffered from **upper respiratory tract** symptoms including sore throat, fever and headache, and then went to the pharmacy to buy some anti-inflammatory drugs. He took six to eight tablets a day and the symptoms relieved quickly after 3 days. Yesterday morning, he found some numbness feeling on his feet when standing or walking, and swellings around his ankles after sitting and writing calligraphy for about two hours. He did not have similar experience before and was very worried about it. The next day, the worsening condition of numbness and swelling made him visit our clinic for help.

Past History:

1. DM for 15 years; renal insufficiency for 5 years.

2. Admission about once per year for the past three years, for the purpose of blood sugar control.

3. No operation history.

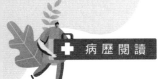
Personal History:

1. Medication: Amaryl 3# QD, Acarbose 1# TID with first bite of meals.

2. Alcohol(-), betel nut(-), smoking (1 **PPD** for more than 30 years).

3. Allergic history: No drug or food allergy.

Family History:

1. Mother: DM for 20 years, died of **ARF** at 50 years old.

2. All of his siblings have poorly controlled blood sugar.

Review of System:

Mild dyspnea in climbing more than 2 flights of stairs, no symptoms related to other organ systems.

Physical Examination:

1. General appearance: Anxious. BP: 150/96 mmHg, PR: 96/min, RR: 20/min.

2. Conjunctiva: Not anemic, sclera: Not icteria.

3. Neck: Supple; no jugular vein engorgement; no palpable lymph node; normal sized thyroid gland; no carotid bruit.

4. Chest: Symmetric expansion; faint crackles could be heard all over bilateral lung bases.

5. Heart: Regular heart beats; no murmur; normal S_1 and S_2, no S_3 or S_4.

6. Abdomen: Slight globular; no tenderness or rebound tenderness; no mass palpable, no hepatosplenomegaly.

7. Extremities: No deformity; free joint movement. Bilateral lower legs and ankles pitting edema.

8. Mild loss of light touch and pinprick sensation on both feet, no sign of muscle weakness.

Impression:

1. Diabetic mellitus, suspected diabetic **neuropathy** and **nephropathy**.

2. Dyspnea and edema of undefined cause.

Management:

1. Arrange urine dipstick test, blood tests including complete blood count, biochemistry, and **electrocardiogram**.

2. Diet salt (sodium) restriction.

3. Furosemide 40 mg/tab 1# QD PO.

4. Return to clinic two days later.

Attending Physician: ×××

關鍵字彙 Keywords

字　彙	原　文	中　譯
Numbness		麻痺
DM	diabetes mellitus	糖尿病
Upper respiratory tract		上呼吸道
PPD	pack per day	每日幾包（菸）
ARF	acute renal failure	急性腎衰竭
Neuropathy	neuro-，神經 -pathy，病變	神經病變
Nephropathy	nephro-，腎臟	腎病變
Electrocardiogram	electro-，電 -cardio-，心臟 -gram，圖、攝影	心電圖
Hypoglycemic	hypo-，低、不足 -gly，糖 -emic，血	低血糖

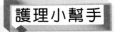
護理小幫手

Little Helper

認識急性腎衰竭

急性腎衰竭是指腎臟突然失去功能，通常急性腎衰竭依其原因可分為腎前性(pre-renal)、腎因性(intrinsic renal)及腎後性(post-renal)三大類。腎前性是因為灌流不足所造成，例如：脫水、心臟衰竭、肝硬化等；腎因性是指除了灌流不足以外的因素，例如：敗血症、有腎毒性的藥物及顯影劑等；腎後性是指泌尿系統阻塞所引致。其症狀會有發燒、噁心、嘔吐、水腫、高血壓、呼吸喘、頭痛、痙攣、昏睡、昏迷等。此時需注意維持水分及電解質的平衡，若有感染時需使用抗生素；有高血壓患者，必須控制血壓，避免因高血壓引發腎衰竭；飲食控制需採高熱量、低蛋白飲食減少代謝廢物產生，並限制鈉及鉀食物攝取；適當的休息，以免疲勞過度。

Follow-Up Visit

2023-2-7　　10:40 a.m.

Chief Complaints and Problems:

1. Bilateral lower legs and ankles swelling, slightly improved.

2. Feet numbness persists.

3. Exertional dyspnea progressed.

Physical Examination:

1. BP: 148/86 mmHg, PR: 84/min, RR: 16/min.

2. Pitting edema at lower legs and ankles less than before.

3. Bilateral crackle breath sounds with less prominence.

Laboratory data:

1. CBC

Date	RBC	Platelet	Hb	WBC	MCV
2023-2-5	3.40 M/uL	290,500/μL	11.2 g/dL	6,500/μL	92.5 fL

2. BCS

Date	Glucose (AC)	BUN	Creatinine	ALT	Sodium	Potassium
2023-2-5	180 mg/dL	67 mg/dL	9.5 mg/L	40 U/L	129 mEq/L	6.2 mEq/L

3. Urine dipstick

Date	Protein	Sugar	Occult blood	WBC
2023-2-5	+++	++	+	++

4. Electrocardiogram: Sinus tachycardia and ST segment depression (V3 to V6).

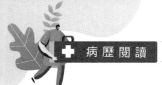

Diagnosis:

1. Diabetes mellitus.

2. Acute exacerbation of chronic renal failure.

3. Suspected urinary tract infection.

4. Suspected drug-induced nephropathy.

5. Suspected ischemic heart disease.

Management:

1. Continue diuretic treatment and diet modification.

2. Modified diabetic treatment, discontinue oral **hypoglycemic** agents and start insulin treatment.

3. Arrange admission for further evaluation and treatment.

Attending Physician: ×××

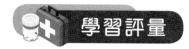 學習評量

一、選擇題

( )1. 下列腎衰竭症狀中，何者並非此個案的症狀？(A)numbness of feet (B)swelling of ankles (C)breathing sound clear (D)dyspnea

( )2. 下列何者可能是此個案引發腎衰竭的危險因素？(A)hypertension (B)drug-induced nephropathy (C)hyperlipidemia (D)smoking

( )3. 下列何種飲食較適合腎衰竭的病人？(A)low calorie diet (B)high protein diet (C)low salt diet (D)high potassium diet

( )4. 下列何者並非個案在複診時出現的身體症狀？(A)兩側小腿與足踝水腫更嚴重 (B)足部麻木感持續 (C)心搏過快 (D)呼吸困難加劇

( )5. 請問此個案所出現的水腫屬於下列哪一種？(A)lymphedema (B)epidermal edema (C)myxedema (D)pitting edema

二、填充題

請寫出以下縮寫或生字之全文及中譯。

1. Numbness_____

2. Pittingedema_____

3. Neuropathy_____

4. Nephropathy_____

5. Electrocardiogram_____

6. Dyspnea_____

7. Urinarytractinfection_____

8. ARF_____

學習評量解答
請掃描 QR Code

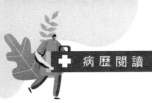
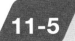

11-5 Rehabilitation

Initial Visit

2023-4-30   10:30 a.m.

Source of Information:

Patient herself.

Chief Complaint:

Aggravated lower back pain for two weeks.

Present Illness:

There is a 55 year-old woman experiencing chronic **lower back pain** for one year. She had received medication and physical therapies at local clinic off and on. Two weeks ago, she began to have lower back pain after bending forward to take a heavy object from the floor. Therefore, she received **physical therapy** and medication at a local clinic for one week, but the pain continued. She then received three sessions of **needle acupuncture** treatment at a Traditional Chinese Medicine clinic. However, progressive intractable lower back pain with radiation to the right lower leg developed since three days ago, so that she could not sit, stand, or walk. Therefore, she was brought to our hospital by her husband for further evaluation. Cough, sneezing and defecation would aggravate the right sciatic pain, and bed rest could improve the pain mildly.

Past History:

1. Peptic ulcer with bleeding two years ago.
2. Denied cardiac, renal, or hepatic disease.
3. Denied drinking.
4. Denied smoking.
5. Post surgical history: Myoma s/p hysterectomy at 10 years ago.

Family History:

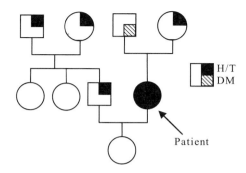

H/T
DM

Patient

Medication Allergy History:

No known medication allergy.

Travel History:

Denied having gone to abroad in recent half year.

Occupation and Work Status:

Housewife.

Review of System:

Musculoskeletal system: Lower back pain(+), right sciatic pain(+).

No symptoms related to other organ systems.

Physical Examination:

1. Body height: 160 cm, body weight: 60 kg, blood pressure: 122/84 mmHg.
2. Neck: Supple, no lymph node palpable, no JVE.
3. Chest: Symmetric expansion, BS: Clear.
4. Heart: Regular HR, no murmur.
5. Abdomen: Soft and flat, no tenderness, no rebound pain, no abnormal mass palpable.

6. Standing with rigid spine. Severe muscle spasm over back. Tenderness over lower back(+). Knocking pain over lower back(-).

7. Flexion: Failed due to pain.

   Extension: Failed due to pain.

   Rotation: Failed due to pain.

   Endurance for sit, stand, and walk: Poor, less than a few min.

   SLRT: 30 degrees/60 degrees, crossed over left side.

   Muscle strength:

   Hip flexor: Normal/normal.

   Knee extensor: Normal/normal.

   Ankle dorsiflexor: Fair(+) grade/normal.

   EHL: Fair(+) grade/normal.

   Ankle plantarflexor: Normal/normal.

   Sensation: Decreased light touch and pin prick over right dorsal foot and big toe.

   DTR:

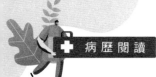

   Sphincter: Continent to stool and bladder.

Diagnosis:

Herniated intervertebral disc with right sciatic pain.

Management:

1. Lumbar spine AP and lateral views.

2. NSAIDs and muscle relaxant.

3. Bed rest for 2 days.

4. Local ice packing.

5. Patient education for postural correction.

Make appointment:

Follow up 3 days later.（預約 5 月 3 日回診）

Attending Physician: ×××

護理小幫手

Little Helper

何謂 SLRT？

　　直立抬腿測驗(straight leg raising test, SLRT)主要測驗 L3 以下高度有神經根受壓迫的狀況。測試時，先讓病人仰臥、放輕鬆，下肢伸直。測試者以一手置於病人腳跟下方，慢慢抬高，當病人出現疼痛現象表示坐骨神經受到壓迫。若抬高的角度小於 70 度有疼痛加劇的現象，表示 L5 或 S1 可能受壓迫；當腿部伸直抬舉並在腳掌背屈時疼痛加劇時，稱 Bragard's test(＋)；當屈膝時疼痛緩減，但膝蓋若伸直卻使疼痛加劇，此為 Lasegue's test(＋)。

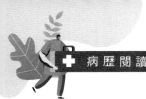

關鍵字彙 Keywords

字　彙	原　文	中　譯
Lower back pain		下背痛
Physical therapy		物理治療
Needle acupuncture		針灸
SLRT	straight leg raising test	直立抬腿測驗
EHL	extensor hallucis longus	伸拇長肌
DTR	deep tendon reflex	深肌腱反射
HIVD	Herniated intervertebral disc	椎間盤突出症

護理小幫手

Little Helper

認識椎間盤突出症

　　椎間盤若受到突然的重力或長期承受壓力，周圍的韌帶因此受損或弱化，則髓核由韌帶間突出，壓迫到脊髓或推移脊神經，稱為椎間盤突出症，以第 4 與 5 腰椎間、第 5 腰椎、第 1 薦椎間(L4~L5、L5~S1)最常見。

　　椎間盤突出是下背痛的主要原因，疼痛會因咳嗽、用力、久坐、久站而加劇。深部肌腱反射可能會變弱（深腱反射的評分是 0~4 分：0＝無反射、1＝減弱、2＝正常、3＝增加、4＝過度）、患側神經所管轄的區域感覺遲鈍。診斷性檢查方面可從脊髓 X 光攝影發現脊椎退化，但看不出腰椎間盤是否破裂；直立抬腿測驗腿舉至 30 度以上時，產生神經痛。

　　治療上可採椎板切除術、藥物治療（止痛劑、抗炎症反應劑、抗痙攣劑、肌肉鬆弛劑、鎮靜劑）、物理治療〔深部超音波熱療法、熱敷、牽引、背部肌肉運動（仰臥起坐、骨盆抬高、膝胸運動）〕。

Follow-Up Visit

2023-5-3   10:40 a.m.

S: Mild improvement of lower back pain with right lower limb radiation pain after medication and bed rest for 3 days.

O: Lumbar spine AP and lateral views show: Disc space narrowing at level of L4/L5.

Standing with a rigid spine.

Flexion: Mild limitation due to pain.

Extension: Mild limitation due to pain.

Rotation: To right: Mild limitation due to pain; to left: Full range.

SLRT: 65 degrees/90 degrees.

Endurance for sit: Improving to 20 min.

Endurance for stand: Improving to 10 min.

Endurance for walk: Improving to 5 min.

Muscle strength:

Hip flexor: Normal/normal.

Knee extensor: Normal/normal.

Ankle dorsiflexor: Fair(+) grade/normal.

EHL: Fair(+) grade/normal.

Ankle plantarflexor: Normal/normal.

A: HIVD with right sciatic pain, suspect right L5 **radiculopathy**.

P:

1. Arrange **pelvic traction** followed by local hot pack, **TENS** over lower back and right lower limb.

2. Patient education for postural correction and home program for back muscle stretch and strengthening exercise.

3. Continue present medication.

4. Arrange **electrodiagnostic** study, including **NCV** and **EMG** study.

5. Follow up at 2 weeks later.

Attending Physician: ×××

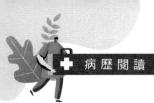

 關鍵字彙 Keywords

字　彙	原　文	中　譯
Radiculopathy	-pathy，病變	神經根病變、神經痛
Pelvic traction		骨盆腔牽引
TENS	transcutaneous electrical nerve stimulation	經皮神經電刺激
Electrodiagnostic	electro-，電	神經電學檢查
NCV	nerve conduction velocity	神經傳導速度
EMG	electromyography	肌電圖

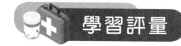

一、選擇題

( )1. 下列何者並非本個案發生 HIVD 的典型症狀？(A)lower back pain (B)muscle spasm over back (C)SLRT 30 to 60 degrees (D)DTR+++

( )2. 下列何者為本個案病史？(A)peptic ulcer (B)COPD (C)AF (D)MR

( )3. 請問個案受損的脊神經位於第幾段？(A)C5 (B)L4 (C)L5 (D)S1

( )4. 下列何者為個案複診時的身體檢查結果？(A)Knocking pain over lower back(+) (B)SLRT: 30 degrees/60 degrees (C)Muscle strength abnormal (D)Standing with rigid spine

( )5. 下列何者並非醫師安排的物理治療方法個案？(A)pelvic traction (B)ultrasound therapy (C)postural correction (D)TENS

二、填充題

請寫出以下縮寫或生字之全文及中譯。

1. Radiculopathy_____

2. Musclestrength_____

3. Lowerbackpain_____

4. Needleacupuncture_____

5. Pelvictraction_____

6. TENS_____

7. HIVD_____

8. DTR_____

9. EHL_____

10. SLRT_____

學習評量解答
請掃描 QR Code

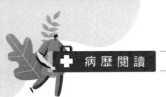
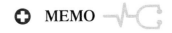 MEMO

12 | CHAPTER

老年醫學病歷

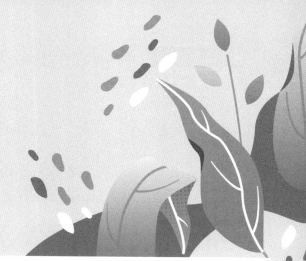

作者｜張皓翔

Admission Note

Geriatric Functional Review

☑ **閱讀導引**

1. 了解病人主訴與現在病史的關係。

2. 分析現在病史與過去病史之關聯性。

3. 分析現在病史、檢驗值與治療措施的合適性。

☑ **PREVIEW**

閱讀本章前，請讀者先自行預習老人疾病相關知識喔！

1. 老年醫學科病例記錄重點。

2. 老年病症的評估與診斷方式。

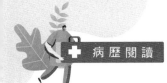

Admission Note

Geriatrics, Female, 82 years old, merried.

Source of information: The patient.

Chief Complaint:

Progressive weight loss 6 kg in 6 months.

Present Illness:

This is a 82 year-old lady with the following medical conditions.

1. **Rheumatoid arthritis**, on hydroxychloroquine 200 mg BID (Plaquenil), methotrexate 10 mg QW, celecoxib 100 mg QD (Celebrex), and folic acid 5 mg BID.

   註：藥品的記錄應以學名為主，並載明劑量及使用頻率，其商品名也可於病歷中註明。

2. **Rheumatic heart disease** with severe aortic stenosis & regurgitation, mitral stenosis & regurgitation, status post **AVR** + **MVR** + **TVR** on 2010/06/25, on furosemide 40 mg QD (Lasix), digoxin 0.25 mg QD (Lanoxin), warfarin 2.5 mg QD (Cofarin).

3. Chronic anemia, suspected hemorrhoid bleeding related, on oral iron supplement.

4. Asthma, on Seretide 1 puff QD~BID (salmeterol 25 mcg + fluticasone 50 mcg/puff), acetylcysteine 600 mg BID (Actein).

5. Constipation, on MgO 250 mg QID.

6. Insomnia.

7. Lung tumor, right upper lobe, with regularly follow-up.

She lives with her husband and children in an apartment with elevators, and her ADL is total independent. She's regularly visited some cardiologist, chest specialist, proctologist and rheumatologist for the above mentioned medical conditions.

She mentioned that slightly decreased oral intake had been noted right after she visited a doctor for rheumatoid arthritis and started to take medications 1 year ago. She was transferred to another rheumatologist because she felt non-satisfactory rapport with that rheumatologist. Hydroxychloroquine, methotrexate, Celebrex, and folic acid had been given to her. However, the condition progressed to poor appetite (reduced to <30% as baseline) with weight loss about 6 kg in the past 6 months since visiting the new rheumatologist. She emphasized that it was "methotrexate" to be the culprit. Even the rheumatologist didn't agree with her and her symptoms of arthritis were improving, she still suspended methotrexate for 2 weeks. In addition, she also noted dizziness with weakness and unsteady gait in the past 6 months. She had intermittent lower gastrointestinal bleeding due to hemorrhoid for over 20 years with chronic anemia. She denied fever, headache, nausea/vomiting, chest tightness, respiratory symptoms, urinary symptoms, or diarrhea. However, intermittent right lower abdominal dull pain without radiation and **tenesmus** was also noted.

Because of above-mentioned symptoms, she went to a geriatrician. In visiting, her vital signs were stable. Physical examination showed pale conjunctiva, clear breath sound, irregular heart beat with systolic murmur, normoactive bowel sound, soft abdomen with RLQ slight tenderness without peritoneal sign, no flank knocking pain, freely movable extremities without edema or rash. Neurological examination showed no focal neurologic deficit, clear consciousness, full/symmetric muscle power, mild unsteady gait. Review of lab data showed normal white count, microcytic anemia (hemoglobin: 7.6 gm/dL), elevated C-reactive protein (1.84), normal liver/kidney function, no electrolyte imbalance. The chest X film showed cardiomegaly, and no active lung lesion. ECG showed atrial fibrillation. Under the impression of unintentional weight loss (6 kg in 6 months) and associated complicated medical conditions, she was admitted for comprehensive geriatric assessment.

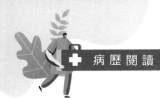
> **病歷小幫手**
>
> Little Helper
>
> 　　過去病史也可以是現在病史，可以在 past history 中呈現，因為同時也是現存慢性醫療問題，在老年醫學評估中是很重要的一環，所以放在 present illness 中一併呈現：風濕性關節炎；風溼性心臟病；慢性貧血，疑痔瘡出血所致；氣喘；便祕；失眠；肺腫瘤，右上肺葉。

Past History:

1. Systemic disease: As above.

2. Hospitalization and surgical history:
   Mixed hemorrhoid, status post hemorrhoidectomy in 2003/11.
   Neuroma, left ulnar, status post excision in 2004/07.

3. Allergy history:
   Indomethacin (Methacin Gel 1% 20 g/tube) Skin rash（皮膚疹）
   Bromelain 20,000 U + L-cysteine 20 mg (Broen-C Enteric F.C./tab)（喘）
   Montelukast Sodium (Singulair 10 mg/tab) Skin rash (hand)

4. Current medication:
   Hydroxychloroquine 200 mg BID
   Methotrexate 10 mg QW
   Celecoxib 100 mg QD
   Folic acid 5 mg BID
   Furosemide 40 mg QD
   Digoxin 0.25 mg QD
   Warfarin 2.5mg QD
   Ferrous fumarate 50 mg BID
   Seretide 1 puff QD~BID (Salmeterol 25 mcg + Fluticasone 50 mcg/puff)
   Acetylcysteine 600 mg BID
   MgO 250 mg QID

5. Travel history: No recent travel.

6. Occupation: housewife.

7. Contact and cluster history: Nil.

8. Family history: Hypertension (father, mother, sisters), Pancreatic cancer (Mom), Parkinson's disease (Brother), Sjögren syndrome (Sister).

9. OBS/GYN history:

G3P3 (NSD*3), marital status: Married.

Menarche: 13 years old, menopause at the age of 46, hormone therapy: Nil.

Last Pap smear and result: Not performed before

Psychosocial Assessment:

教育程度：高中

宗教信仰：佛教

婚姻狀態：已婚

使用語言：國語、台語

口述血型：A，RH：未知，輸血反應：沒輸過血

吸菸：沒有

喝酒：沒有

檳榔：沒有

物質濫用：沒有

Psychological History and Evaluation:

意識狀態：警醒

認知功能：正常

精神情緒狀態：異常、焦慮

安全問題：無

睡眠形態：異常，淺、易醒

Nutritional Screen:

攝食情形：差，攝食 50%以下

排便狀態：異常

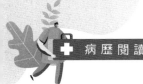
排便異常狀態：便祕

BMI: 18.19

Review of Systems:

1. Systemic: Fever(-), Weight loss (+, 5 kg for 6 months), easy-fatigability(-), change of appetite (+, <30% as baseline), dizziness(+).（註：針對系統性回顧中出現 "+" 的症狀與徵候適當說明）

2. Skin: Petechiae(-), purpura(-), itching(-), local redness and swelling(-), papules(-).

3. HEENT: Hearing loss(-), nasal discharge(-), sore throat(-) headache(-).

4. Cardiovascular: Palpitation(-), exertional dyspnea(-).

5. Respiratory: Dyspne(-), chest pain(-), cough(-).

6. GI: Anorexia(-), nausea(-), vomiting(-), constipation(+), diarrhea(-), melena(-), change of bowel habit(-), small caliber of stool(-), tenesmus (+, for a long period), flatulence(-), abdominal pain (+, RLQ, dull), hematochezia (+, intermittent post defecation).

7. Urogenital: Flank soreness(-), hematuria(-), urinary frequency(-), urgency(-), dysuria(-), hesitancy(-), nocturia(-), polyuria(-), oliguria(-).

8. Musculoskeletal: Back pain(-), bone pain(-), joint pain(-).

Physical Examination:

1. Height: 150.5 cm, Weight: 41.2 kg, Body mass index: 18.12.

2. T: 36.4 °C, Pulse Rate: 90 bpm, R: 16 /min, BP: 112 / 66 mmHg.

3. Pain score: 0.

4. HEENT: Grossly normal, conjunctiva: pale, sclera: anicteric.
   Pupil: Isocoric, 3 mm/3 mm; Light reflex: L/R: +/+; EOM: full and free.

5. Neck: Supple, LAP(-) Goiter(-) Carotid bruit(-).

6. Chest: Symmetric expansion, breath sounds: clear.

7. Heart: Irregular HB, systolic murmur.

8. Abdomen: Soft and flat, bowel sound: normoactive.

9. Liver/spleen: Impalpable; Tenderness (+, RLQ), Rebound tenderness(-).

10. Back: No flank knocking tenderness.

11. Extremities: Freely movable, Pitting edema(-); Cyanosis(-).

12. Skin: Skin rash(-).

13. Peripheral pulsation: Intact.

Brief Neurological Examination:

1. Consciousness: Clear.

2. Muscle power: Full and symmetric.

3. Gait: Mild unsteady.

Neurological Examination:

1. Consciousness: Clear, E4M6V5.

2. Cranial nerve:
   - I   Not checked.
   - II   VA: As baseline; VF (by confrontation test): Intact.
             Pupil size: 3 mm/3 mm, LR: +/+.
   - III, IV, VI   Ptosis(-), retraction(-), Horner syndrome(-). EOM: Intact.
   - V   Corneal reflex: R / L= +/ +.
             Sensory: Facial skin sensation: intact.
             Motor: Jaw movement: no deviation.
   - VII   No facial palsy.
   - VIII   Hearing impairment: Right(-), left(-). Rinne test: Right AC>BC,
             left AC>BC;
             Weber test: no deviation. Nystagmus: Nil.
   - IX, X Gag reflex: R / L = +/+; Soft palate movement: Symmetric.
   - XI   SCM / Trapezius muscle: No weakness.
   - XII   Tongue protrusion: No atrophy, fasciculation or deviation of
             tongue.

3. Motor system:
   - Muscle status: Hypertrophy(-), atrophy(-), fasciculation(-).
   - Muscle tone: No spasticity or flaccidity.
   - Muscle power: Intact muscle power of four limbs.
   - Deep tendon reflex: Normoreflexia in four limbs.

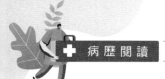

- Pathological reflex: Babinski sign(-), extensor plantar response / flexor plantar response.（extensor 為異常）
- Hoffmann sign (-/-), Glabellar reflex (-/-), Palmomental reflex (-/-).

4. Sensory system:
   - Pinprick: Intact.
   - Temperature: Intact.
   - Vibration: Intact.
   - Joint position sensation: Intact.
   - Double simultaneous stimulation test: No hemineglect.
   - Graphesthesia, stereognosis: Intact.

5. Vestibular system and coordination:
   - Finger-nose-finger: No dysmetria or dysdiadochokinesia.
   - Heel-knee-shin: No dysmetria or dysdiadochokinesia.
   - RAM-no bradykinesia or dysdiadochokinesia.
   - Romberg sign(-).
   - Gait: Mild unsteady.
   - Extrapyramidal system: Rigidity(-), rest tremor(-), bradykinesia(-), loss of postural reflex(-).

6. Autonomic system:
   - Anal sphincter tone: Intact.
   - Urethra sphincter tone: Intact.
   - Postural hypotension(-).
   - Hyper- or hypohidrosis(-).

7. Mental state and high cortical function:
   - Attention: Digit forward and digit backward: intact.
   - Judgement: Intact.
   - Orientation: Person(v), place(v), time(v).
   - Memory: 3-object test: registry: intact; recall: intact.
   - Abstract thinking: Intact.
   - Calculation: Series 7: intact.
   - Speech: Fluency, comprehension, repetition, naming, reading, and writing: intact.

關鍵字彙 Keywords

字 彙	原 文	中 譯
Rheumatoid arthritis		類風濕性關節炎
Rheumatic heart disease		風濕性心臟病
AVR	aortic valve replacement	主動脈瓣置換術
MVR	mitral valve replacement	二尖瓣置換術
TVRL	tricuspid valve replacement	三尖瓣置換術
Tenesmus		裡急後重
TOCC	T: travel history 旅遊史 O: occupation 職業 C: contact history 接觸史 C: cluster history 群聚史	TOCC 資料在發燒或疑似流行病的病人，一定要仔細詢問

Laboratory:

1. Hemogram

WBC	RBC	Hb	Hct	MCV	MCH	MCHC	PLT
3.15 k/uL	3.57 M/μL	7.6 g/dL	27.5 %	77.0 fL	30.7 pg	28.7 g/dL	77 k/uL

Seg	Eos	Baso	Mono	Lym
73.3%	4.8%	0.3%	7.0%	14.6%

2. General BioChemistry

ALT	CRE	Na	K	Alb
27 U/L	1.6 mg/dL	139 mmol/L	5.2 mmol/L	3.7 gm/dL

3. EKG: Atrial fibrillation

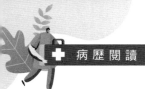

Geriatric Functional Review

<<u>DEEPIN</u>>

Delirium: Confusion Assessment Method (CAM):

 (-) 1. Acute onset with fluctuation.

 (-) 2. Inattention.

 (-) 3. Disorganized thinking.

 (-) 4. Altered level of consciousness.

Depression:

 Depressed mood(+), Loss of interest(-) Suicidal ideation (within 2 weeks) (-)

 <u>GDS</u>-4 (+): 2.

 GDS-15 (+): 6.

Dementia：

 Mini-Cog:

  3-item registration (3/3).

  Clock drawing test (not test).

  3-item recall (3/3).

 MMSE (30)：國中畢業，國語台語，可讀寫(20××/××/××)

  A：現在××年××月××日 星期×(4/4)

   地方：××市，××醫院(2/2)

  B：3 item registration（三個物品短期記憶）：紅色，快樂，腳踏車(3/3)

  C：100 減 7：93(v) 86(v) 79(v) 72(v) 65(v) (5/5)

  D：3 item recall：紅色，快樂，腳踏車(3/3)

  E：這是什麼：錶、筆(2/2)

   覆誦：白紙真正寫黑字(1/1)

   覆讀理解：請閉上眼睛(1/1)

   書寫造句：謝謝大家(1/1)

   口語理解及行動能力：用左手拿紙、摺起來、交給我(3/3)

   圖形抄繪：(1/1)

Eyes: Uncorrected visual impairment affects daily activity(-).

Ears: Uncorrected hearing impairment affects daily activity(-).

Physical performance: Functional decline within 1 year.

    ADL (100/100).

    IADL (8/8).

    Falls: $\geq$1 fall(s) in 1 year(-).

Polypharmacy: $\geq$8 (+, 12).

Pain: VAS 3/10.

Pressure sore: Nil.

Incontinence: Urinary(-), Fecal(-).

Iatrogenesis: NG(-), foley(-), tracheostomy(-), restraint(-), others(-).

Nutrition: BMI $\leq$ 18.5(+, 18.2), BMI $\geq$ 27(-), weight loss 5% in 1 month/10% in 6 months (+, 5 kg), albumin less than 3.5 g/dL(-), swallowing/feeding problem(-).

High health care utilization: Admission$\geq$2/year(-), ER visits$\geq$2/year(-).

DNR: Discussed(-), Accepted(-).

Caregiver issue: Main caregiver: husband; Decision maker: herself.

Socioeconomic issues : Live alone(-), economic problem(-).

Family conference : Need to be arranged(-).

Others: Nil.

<Frailty Screening>

1. **Clinical Frailty Scale**: 3/9.

2. **Tentative Diagnosis**:

    (1) Unintentional weight loss and multi-factor related frailty.

    (2) Renal insufficiency.

3. Underlying chronic illness.

    (1) Rheumatoid arthritis.

    (2) Rheumatic heart disease with severe aortic stenosis & regurgitation, mitral stenosis & regurgitation, status post AVR + MVR + TVR.

    (3) Chronic anemia, suspected hemorrhoid bleeding related.

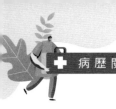

(4) Asthma, stable.

(5) Constipation, stable.

(6) Insomnia.

(7) Lung tumor, right upper lobe, with regularly follow-up.

Plans:

1. Check possible physical conditions that may lead to weight loss, including uncontrolled diabetes, thyroid function, and malignancy.

2. Check the causes of deteriorated renal function.

3. Correct geriatric syndrome related conditions including poor nutritional status, polypharmacy, depressed mood as the geriatric assessment.

Nutritional Condition by Dietician:

-Problem: Underweight.

-Etiology：長時間熱量及高生理價蛋白質食物攝取不足。

-Signs/Symptoms: BMI<18.5.

鼓勵進食，採少量多餐（定時用餐）飲食方式，含纖營養補充品目標 500 kcal／天。增加高生理價蛋白質食物種類及來源，如魚、肉類或選擇蛋、豆製品及營養補充品。增加飲食中油脂（植物油）的攝取量，如以煎、炒取代清燙或水煮。

Polypharmacy:

Avoid iatrogenic medical use, discuss with rheumatologist and cardiologist for the flexibility of medicine reduction.

Depressed Mood:

Support the patient and family, treat underlying disease, consult psychologist or psychiatrist, give anti-depressant if necessary.

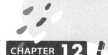
 關鍵字彙 Keywords

字　彙	原　文	中　譯
DEEPIN	D: dementia, depression, delirium E: eye problems, ear problems P: physical performance, polypharmacy, pain, pressure sore I: incontinence, iatrogensis N: nutrition	常見老年病症候群以 DEEPIN 口訣來列表
GDS	Geriatric Depression Scale	老年憂鬱量表。GDS-4 簡式 4 題，作為篩檢用；GDS-15 完整 15 題，每題 1 分。5 分以下為正常，超過 6 分以上應進一步評估憂鬱
Mini-Cog	Mini-Cognitive Assessment Instrument	迷你認知功能測驗。認知功能先以 mini-cog 3-irem recall, serial 7 來評估，如出現問題則應照會神經科醫師，或由有經驗的醫療人員進行 MMSE 的評估
MMSE	Mini-Mental State Examination	簡短心智評估量表，須由專業人員進行評估，判讀需依據病患的教育程度、原本的智能狀態等因素綜合評估
ADL	activities of daily living	日常生活活動評估，一般以巴氏量表(Barthel index)來評估，0~20 分為完全依賴、21~60 分為嚴重依賴、61~90 分為中度依賴、91~99 分為輕度依賴、100 分為完全獨立
IADL	instrumental activities of daily living	用來評估病人獨立自主在社會上生活的能力，包括準備食物、購物、維持家務、打電話、管理財務、就醫、外出交通等，一般以 Lawton 和 Brody 研發的量表評估

字　彙	原　文	中　譯
Clinical Frailty Scale		臨床衰弱量表由 Dalhousie University 發展出來，將老人衰弱程度分為 1~9 級，以圖示來輔助評估，簡明扼要。其他衰弱量表 Kihon check list 以及 Lnda Fried 或 Rockwood 等人模式也經常被使用
Tentative diagnosis		臆斷依據目前病況與檢查所作的初步診斷，未必是最終診斷，可能因近一步的檢查有所發現而改變

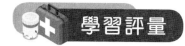 學習評量

一、選擇題

( )1. 以下何者不是病人主要的入院原因？(A) Rheumatic heart disease (B) Weight loss (C) Poor appetite (D) Dizziness and weakness

( )2. 請問病人的個人病史中下列何者為是？(A) Increased oral take (B) Weight loss about 6 kg in the past 6 months (C) Chest pain since one week ago (D) Fever for one day

( )3. 常見老年病徵候群以什麼口訣評估？(A)DEEPIN (B)IADL (C)MMSE (D)ADL

( )4. 病人的系統性評估與身體檢查方面，下列何者為是？(A) Skin rash (+) (B) Depressed mood (+) (C) Clouding of consciousness (D) Goiter(+)

( )5. 下列何項非病人現在服用的藥物？(A) Folic acid (B) Hydroxychloroquine (C) Methotrexate (D) Celebrex

二、填充題

請寫出以下縮寫或生字之全文及中譯。

1. Tenesmus _____

2. Mini-Cog _____

3. MMSE _____

4. Rheumatoid arthritis _____

5. TOCC 的 T _____

學習評量解答
請掃描 QR Code

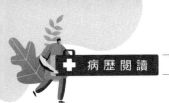

MEMO

13 | CHAPTER

護理記錄

作者 | 潘昭貴

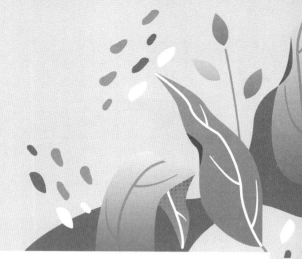

☑ 閱讀導引

1. 了解記錄的意義與目的。
2. 了解書寫記錄時的原則有哪些。
3. 了解護理記錄的重要性。
4. 認識各種護理記錄表單格式及其使用時機。

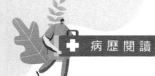

13-1 記錄概述

記錄的意義與目的

　　記錄(record)是指「將某段時間所發生的事實記載下來」；而醫療記錄(medical record)及病歷記錄則是指專業的醫療小組成員根據病人的診斷，或是在某段時間內與病人之間的互動，包括觀察、護理及治療等情形，依實際發生的現況，以有效、具體的文字呈現。

　　記錄在醫療照護上極為重要，其目的在於提供溝通、教學參考、評估、研究參考、審核、法律證明文件、提供醫療費用償還與給付證明，其中以「提供溝通」為最主要的目的。

　　書寫記錄時需掌握以下原則：真實性、精確性、完整性、時效性、組織性、統一性及簡潔扼要。

1. **真實性**：真的有發生的事情、確實有執行的護理照護行為或醫療處置，才能寫在護理記錄上。

　　例如：個案發燒（確有其事）、護理人員確實有衛教個案多喝開水，也依立即醫囑及給予退燒藥，這一連串「有發生之事實」才能記錄在護理記錄上。

2. **精確性**：所謂精確性換言之就是指：「具體」的事實，而此事實最好是可以「量化」、實際描述。

　　例如：(1) 食量差，可以具體說明 → 三餐進食約 1/3 碗稀飯、4~6 口青菜及一湯匙肉末。

　　　　　(2) 解 2 次黑便、量中，可以具體說明 → 解 2 次黑糊便，共約 330 gm。

3. **完整性**：描述事件應由個案現況（主、客觀資料）、護理與醫療處置、衛教及個案於護理、衛教與醫療處置後之反應，全部都要完整敘述。

　　例如：在描述個案傷口時要說明之事項需包括：傷口部位、種類（擦傷、手術傷口、燙傷等）、大小(cm)、顏色、分泌物、氣味、周圍皮膚狀況、患肢末稍血循、傷口護理方式與頻率、衛教之事項、照護與衛教後個案之反應等皆應完整記錄。

4. **時效性**：護理記錄上所寫的時間點為「事件發生的時間」，所以書寫護理記錄應在事件發生後立即記錄才具時效性，也可以預防忘記事件發生的時間或因護理工作繁忙而忘了記錄該事件。

5. **組織性**：在書寫護理記錄時要注意其組織性，可以按各系統書寫或由頭至腳描述，勿雜亂無章地書寫。

　　例如：　在記錄有關個案 N-G feeding 的消化情形，可以這樣書寫 → N-G tube 固定於 60 cm 處，Q4H 灌食 300 mL，消化情形良好，聽診腸蠕動：8~11次／分，解一次成形黃軟便。

6. **統一性**：書寫護理記錄時的措辭用語要有統一性、一致性，需用醫護人員能理解的共同語言（例如：醫護專有名詞或縮寫）書寫，切勿自行創造新名詞或擅自將英文之醫護專有名詞自創縮寫。

7. **簡潔扼要**：書寫護理記錄宜簡潔扼要，不需要的贅詞就不需要。

　　例如：　傷口紅紅的，有一點點流血及黃色黏黏的分泌物，量中，可以書寫成 → 傷口基底呈紅色，有黃色分泌物，量約滲濕 2×2 吋紗布一塊及滲血量約一元硬幣。

　　　　若已書寫「傷口評估與護理記錄單」就不需重複書寫，護理記錄內容只需寫：詳見傷口評估與護理記錄單。

13-2　護理記錄表單

　　各醫療機構會依機構本身的需求發展出「各類病歷單張」以利醫療團隊可快速、完整、確實有效地完成記錄，以下僅介紹護理病歷、出院護理摘要、傷口評估與護理記錄單、手術前醫囑及護理記錄、手術前病人識別記錄表、排尿訓練記錄表、護理衛教指導表、臨床路徑。

一、護理病歷

1. **記錄時機**：於個案入院時使用。

2. **表單用意**：於個案入院時了解主要入院因素、進行收集個案基本資料、過去病史、長期用藥，並進行初步護理評估時使用。

3. **特殊注意事項**：於護理病歷上已記錄之事項，在護理記錄中不需重複記錄。

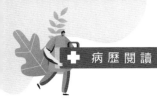
護理病歷

姓名			病歷號碼			床號		科別	
性別	□男 □女		入院日期			時間		年齡	

診斷		資料來源 記錄護理人員	□病人 □親友 □其他＿＿＿＿＿＿

此次 住院 原因	
病史	

生命	體溫：　　℃	呼吸：　　　次／分
徵象	脈搏：　　次／分 □規則 □不規則	血壓：　　　mmHg

入院方式	□門診□急診／□步行□輪椅□推床	主要照顧者	□無 □有／關係：

緊急 聯絡人	姓名：　　　　住家電話：　　　　手機：　　　　與病人關係：

身高	公分	語言	□國語 □台語 □客語 □英語 □原住民語：　　　□其他：
體重	公斤		

溝通能力	□正常 □失語 □構音困難 □無法了解他人所説／所寫 □其他：

過敏	□無 □有／□食物：　　　□藥物：　　　□其他：

GCS	總分：＿＿＿＿（E 、V 、M ）	宗教	□道教□佛教□基督教□天主教□其他＿＿＿
呼吸	□正常□深快□淺快□困難□端坐□喘息 □氣切□插管□輔助器□抽痰□其他＿＿＿＿	教育	□不識字□識字□小學□初中 □高中□大專以上

皮膚	顏色	□正常□蒼白□潮紅□脫皮□乾裂□其他	身分	□健保□自費□其他＿＿＿＿
	完整性	□完整□不完整（傷口別＿＿＿＿＿＿＿） 部位＿＿＿＿＿＿大小＿＿＿＿＿＿	聽力	左：□正常□重聽□失聰□其他＿＿＿＿ 右：□正常□重聽□失聰□其他＿＿＿＿

檳榔	□無 □有 已吃：＿＿＿年	視力	左：□正常□模糊□失明□偏盲□其他 右：□正常□模糊□失明□偏盲□其他
吸菸	□無 □有，每日：＿＿支、＿＿包，已抽＿＿年	肌力	左上肢：　　　　左下肢： 右上肢：　　　　右下肢：
喝酒	□不喝 □偶喝 □大量 已喝＿＿＿年		

營養狀況	□普通飲食□特殊飲食／飲食類別＿＿＿＿＿ □禁忌：＿＿＿＿＿＿＿＿＿＿＿＿ □由口進食　　□鼻胃管灌食 □腸胃造口　　□其他＿＿＿＿＿＿＿	自我照 顧能力	進食＿＿＿ 穿衣：上身＿＿＿ 下身＿＿＿ 脫衣：上身＿＿＿ 下身＿＿＿ 沐浴＿＿＿ 刷牙＿＿＿ 洗臉＿＿＿ 如廁＿＿＿ 備註：1.完全依賴 2.部分依賴 3.自理

假牙	□無 □有／□固定：□上□下 　　　　　□活動：□上□下	行動	□正常 □無法行動 需輔具：□拐杖 □輪椅 □助行器 □義肢

排泄	小便	□正常 □失禁 □頻尿 □滯留 □尿少 □存留導尿管 □人工造口	疼痛 部位	部位：＿＿＿＿＿＿ 性質：＿＿＿＿＿ 持續時間：＿＿＿＿＿ 止痛藥：□無 □有，藥名：＿＿＿＿＿
	大便	□正常 □失禁 □腹瀉 □便祕 □軟便劑＿＿＿＿＿ □止瀉藥＿＿＿＿＿ □人工肛門	睡眠	＿＿＿小時／天 □正常 □不穩 □失眠 □服用鎮靜（安眠）＿＿＿＿＿＿

二、出院護理摘要

1. **記錄時機**：於個案出院時使用。

2. **表單用意**：於個案出院時作為目前病況摘要說明，並列出出院時仍需持續進行的護理照護問題、各種管路明細及需給予的各項衛教之內容。

3. **特殊注意事項**：於「出院護理摘要」上已記錄之事項，在護理記錄中不需重複記錄。

出院護理摘要

姓名		病歷號碼		床號		科別	
性別	□男 □女	出院日期		時間		年齡	
出院方式	□MBD □AAD □DDT □轉院 □死亡						
返診日期	＿＿年＿＿月＿＿日　上午　下午　＿＿＿＿診／＿＿＿＿號				照會社區	□是 □不需要	
傷口	□無　□有／部位＿＿＿＿＿、類別＿＿＿＿、大小＿＿＿＿				傷口護理	□會 □不會	
診斷書	□不需要　□需要：□甲種診斷書＿＿＿＿份 □乙種診斷書＿＿＿＿份，用途：＿＿＿＿＿＿						
存留管路	□無　□有　□N-G tube（日期：　）　□foley（日期：　）　□氣切（日期：　）　□其他：＿＿＿＿＿＿＿＿（日期：　）						
目前病況摘要							
自我照顧能力	□自理　□需他人協助：□沐浴及個人衛生＿＿＿＿＿＿＿＿　□日常生活照顧＿＿＿＿＿＿＿＿　□其他：＿＿＿＿＿＿＿＿						
護理問題	□已解決　□尚未解決：1.＿＿＿＿＿＿＿＿　2.＿＿＿＿＿＿＿＿　3.＿＿＿＿＿＿＿＿						
出院衛教	□服藥：　□飲食：　□管路：　□活動：　□其他：						
家屬簽名				護理人員簽名			

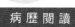

三、傷口評估與護理記錄單

1. **記錄時機**：於評估傷口或進行傷口護理時使用。

2. **表單用意**：方便記錄傷口應進行的各項評估、換藥方式、護理處置及衛教。而且因為「傷口評估與護理記錄單」上的傷口評估項目齊全，有關傷口護理的方式皆有標示，故可提供護理人員傷口照護指引，以協助評估與方便記錄，可減少對於傷口評估不齊全或記錄遺漏之情形發生。

3. **特殊注意事項**：於「傷口評估與護理記錄單」上已記錄之事項，在護理記錄中不需重複記錄，護理記錄內容只需書寫：詳見傷口評估與護理記錄單。

傷口評估與護理記錄單

| 姓名 | | 病歷號碼 | | 床號 | | 性別 □男 □女 | 科別 | |

傷口部位標示圖：（請以筆標示並註明傷口編號）

正面　　　　　　　　　反面

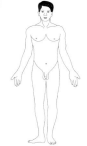 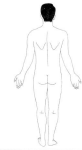

	日期／時間				
傷口評估	傷口編號、部位、等級				
	傷口種類				
	傷口範圍 長×寬×深(cm)				
	傷口基部顏色百分比	完整__ 紅__黃__黑__	完整__ 紅__黃__黑__	完整__ 紅__黃__黑__	完整__ 紅__黃__黑__
	傷口滲出液量	□無□少□中□多	□無□少□中□多	□無□少□中□多	□無□少□中□多
	傷口滲出液性質	□無　　□清澈 □漿液性□血水性 □膿性　□膿血性	□無　　□清澈 □漿液性□血水性 □膿性　□膿血性	□無　　□清澈 □漿液性□血水性 □膿性　□膿血性	□無　　□清澈 □漿液性□血水性 □膿性　□膿血性
	傷口滲出液異味	□有　　□無	□有　　□無	□有　　□無	□有　　□無
傷口護理	換藥次數				
	換藥方式	□生理食鹽水 □水溶性優碘 □透明透氣薄膜 □N/S wet □彈紗　□彈繃 □其他_____	□生理食鹽水 □水溶性優碘 □透明透氣薄膜 □N/S wet □彈紗　□彈繃 □其他_____	□生理食鹽水 □水溶性優碘 □透明透氣薄膜 □N/S wet □彈紗　□彈繃 □其他_____	□生理食鹽水 □水溶性優碘 □透明透氣薄膜 □N/S wet □彈紗　□彈繃 □其他_____
	引流管／種類	□有 □無 □拔除	□有 □無 □拔除	□有 □無 □拔除	□有 □無 □拔除
	傷口細菌培養 感染(＋)、無感染(－)				
	護理處置	□皮膚檢查 □翻身 □減壓裝置／_____ □氣墊床 □抬高患肢 □石膏護理 □其他	□皮膚檢查 □翻身 □減壓裝置／_____ □氣墊床 □抬高患肢 □石膏護理 □其他	□皮膚檢查 □翻身 □減壓裝置／_____ □氣墊床 □抬高患肢 □石膏護理 □其他	□皮膚檢查 □翻身 □減壓裝置／_____ □氣墊床 □抬高患肢 □石膏護理 □其他
	衛教	□傷口注意事項 □換藥	□傷口注意事項 □換藥	□傷口注意事項 □換藥	□傷口注意事項 □換藥
	簽名				

＊傷口編號：依英文字母順序標示(1.2.3……)

＊傷口部位：依右圖數字標示(A.B.C……)，其他部位需註明位置

＊傷口等級：依下列等級標示(Stage I、II、III、IV)

＊傷口種類：A.壓傷　B.術後縫合傷口　C.創傷　D.失禁性皮膚炎　E.其他_____

＊各項評估與護理以「ˇ」表示

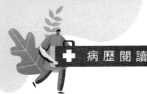

四、手術前醫囑及護理記錄

1. **記錄時機**：於手術前進行醫囑與手術前各項護理使用。

2. **表單用意**：確認手術前應進行的各項醫囑、護理措施與衛教是否已逐項完成，也方便記錄手術前已完成之醫囑、護理與衛教。

3. **特殊注意事項**：於「手術前醫囑與護理記錄單」上已記錄之事項，在護理記錄中不需重複記錄，護理記錄內容只需書寫：詳見手術前醫囑與護理記錄單。

手術前醫護及護理記錄

姓名		病歷號碼		床號		性別	□男 □女	科別	

診斷：

術式：

預定手術時間：＿＿＿年 ＿＿＿月 ＿＿＿日 （上、下）午 ＿＿＿時 ＿＿＿分 或 on call＿＿＿＿＿＿＿

項目	醫囑∨	執行日期	簽名
1	填寫手術同意書		
2	填寫麻醉同意書		
3	皮膚準備－範圍：＿＿＿＿＿＿＿＿＿＿＿＿＿＿＿＿＿		
4	藥物過敏：□無 □有：藥名＿＿＿＿＿＿＿＿＿＿＿＿＿		
5	手術前衛教：(1)深呼吸及有效咳嗽 (2)手術後翻身及早期下床 (3)衛教手術前準備應注意之事項與過程、目的及時間 (4)教導病人或家屬床上使用便盆 (5)教導術後：□傷口 □導管 之照護 (6)其他：＿＿＿＿＿＿＿＿＿＿＿＿＿＿＿＿＿		
6	執行術前病人身體清潔：□洗頭 □洗澡 □其他＿＿＿＿＿＿		
7	追蹤檢查報告：CBC＿＿＿＿、BCS＿＿＿＿、EKG＿＿＿＿、X-Ray＿＿＿＿、其他＿＿＿＿		
8	備血：血型：＿＿＿＿＿＿＿＿＿、 Rh：＿＿＿＿＿＿ Whole Blood＿＿＿＿U、PRBC＿＿＿＿U、FFP＿＿＿＿U、Platelet＿＿＿＿U 其他＿＿＿＿＿＿＿＿＿＿＿＿＿＿＿U		
9	通知禁食（掛禁食時間）：□午夜後 □早餐後 □午餐後 □其他＿＿＿＿＿＿		
10	灌腸：□甘油灌腸 □清潔灌腸 □肥皂水灌腸 □其他＿＿＿＿＿＿＿＿		
11	除去髮夾、假牙、眼鏡、口紅、寇丹、首飾、隱形眼鏡、其他：＿＿＿＿＿＿		
12	更換手術衣、手圈		
13	點滴注射：靜脈留置針＿＿＿＿G ；CVP＿＿＿way、固定＿＿＿cm、部位＿＿＿＿＿ 其他＿＿＿＿＿＿＿＿＿＿＿＿＿＿＿＿＿：部位＿＿＿＿＿＿ 藥物：＿＿＿＿＿＿＿＿＿＿＿＿＿＿＿＿＿＿＿		
14	手術前給藥：＿＿＿＿＿＿＿＿＿＿＿＿＿＿＿＿＿＿＿ 、 給藥時間：＿＿＿＿＿＿＿		
15	手術前□排尿 □導尿：二叉尿管＿＿＿＿Fr. 三叉尿管＿＿＿＿Fr.		
16	生命徵象： BT：＿＿＿℃、PR：＿＿＿次／分、RR：＿＿＿次／分、BP：＿＿＿＿＿＿＿mmHg		
17	攜帶物品：□舊病歷 □藥物：＿＿＿＿＿＿＿＿＿＿＿ □其他：＿＿＿＿＿＿＿		
18	特殊交班事項：		
19	□聯絡家屬（與病人關係：＿＿＿＿＿）並衛教家屬於手術室外等候 □無家屬		
20	送病人至手術室時間：＿＿＿月＿＿＿日 （上、下）午 ＿＿＿時＿＿＿分		

五、手術前病人識別記錄表

1. **記錄時機**：用於手術前進行個案身分確認用。

2. **表單用意**：用於手術前確認個案身分、手術方式及名稱，個案身上標示的手術部位與病歷上的標示部位是否符合；確認地點需包括三處：個案所屬單位（門診、病房、急診或加護病房）、手術等待區及手術室內。

3. **特殊注意事項**：確認地點（個案所屬單位、手術等待區、手術室內）務必確實進行手術前各項確認工作，以防止手術部位錯誤或個案錯誤等無法彌補之醫療疏失。

手術前病人識別記錄表

姓名		病歷號碼		床號		性別	□男　□女	科別	

身分證號：

診斷：

術式：

手術日期、時間：_____年_____月_____日（上、下）午_____時_____分

識別地點：□門診　□病房　□急診　□加護病房　　識別時間：_____	執行醫師簽名與主護簽名

意識清楚	意識不清楚、無法溝通、嬰幼兒	
□核對手圈、病人與病歷符合 □能說出自己姓名、生日 □能說出自己手術方式及部位	□核對手圈、病人、病歷符合 □家屬（與病人之關係：_____）能說出病人姓名、生日 □家屬能說出病人手術方式及部位	

手術部位標示：□未標示　　□已標示：

正面　　　　　　　　　　**反面**

□核對病人手術部位標示與病歷符合

識別地點：手術等待區　　　識別時間：_____	護理人員簽名

□核對手圈、病人與病歷符合 □能說出自己姓名、生日 □能說出自己手術方式及部位	□核對手圈、病人、病歷符合 □家屬（與病人之關係：_____）能說出病人姓名、生日 □家屬能說出病人手術方式及部位	

手術部位標示：□未標示　　□已標示：

正面　　　　　　　　　　**反面**

□核對病人手術部位標示與病歷符合

識別地點：手術室內　　　　識別時間：_____

□核對手圈、病歷與病人符合

□麻醉前確認病人姓名、手術方式及部位

□劃刀前確認病人姓名、手術方式及部位

執行者簽名	手術醫師簽名		麻醉醫師簽名		流動護士簽名	

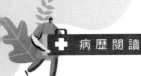

六、排尿訓練記錄表

1. **記錄時機**：用於排尿出現問題，需進行排尿訓練之個案使用。
2. **表單用意**：可運用排尿訓練記錄表上各時間點的飲水量、排尿量、餘尿量，主治醫師可依據上述的數據，進行調整與排尿有關的藥物種類、劑量，護理人員也可依此進行相關排尿的各項衛教。
3. **特殊注意事項**：因為排尿訓練記錄表大多是由個案自己或家屬進行記錄，故每次至病房探視個案時，要適時提醒個案及家屬要記得確實記錄，也需詢問在記錄排尿訓練記錄表時是否有困難，並適時給予協助。

排尿訓練記錄表

| 姓名 | | 病歷號碼 | | | 床號 | | | 性別 | □男 □女 | | 科別 | | |

日期																			
時間	水分	解尿	餘尿	水分	解尿	餘尿	水分	解尿	餘尿	水分	解尿	餘尿	水分	解尿	餘尿				
05:00																			
06:00																			
07:00																			
08:00																			
09:00																			
10:00																			
11:00																			
12:00																			
13:00																			
14:00																			
15:00																			
16:00																			
17:00																			
18:00																			
19:00																			
20:00																			
21:00 On Foley																			
06:00 Remove Foley																			
24hrs Total																			

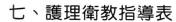

七、護理衛教指導表

1. **記錄時機**：用於進行藥物、身體活動、飲食等護理指導、衛教時使用。

2. **表單用意**：有規劃、有系統地進行護理指導與衛教，而且可清楚了解其進度，並可將已進行護理指導與衛教的事項進行評值，以便確認個案及家屬的了解程度。

3. **特殊注意事項**：有進行護理指導與衛教時一定要確實記錄，若有特殊事項或情況要書寫在護理記錄中並列為交班事項。

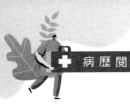
護理衛教指導表

姓名		病歷號碼		床號		性別	□男 □女	科別	

項目	護理指導		指導日期				評值日期			
			/	/	/	/	/	/	/	/
藥物指導	口服藥	種類、_____種 藥物副作用及注意事項 使用時間的遵從性								
	針劑	□大量點滴、藥物副作用及注意事項 □IV、藥物副作用及注意事項 □IM、藥物副作用及注意事項								
	塞劑	藥物副作用及注意事項 □肛門　□陰道								
	其他	□定量噴霧劑使用方法及注意事項								
		□胰島素使用方法及注意事項： 　1.劑量　2.時間　3.部位 　4.無菌　5.抽藥　6.注射方法								
		□其他： 　藥名_____ 　途徑_____								
活動指導	運動重要性與必要性									
	肢體正確的功能性擺位									
	翻身方法與時間、預防關節攣縮									
	運動的禁忌									
	運動方法及注意事項									
	預防跌倒的措施									
	輔助器材的使用及指導									
	其他									
飲食指導	飲食種類：_____									
	飲食的禁忌：_____									
	飲食種類的選擇									
	飲食烹調方法									
	水分攝取的重要性、量：_____c.c.／天									
	管灌飲食：1.注意事項　2.技巧									
	其他									
其他護理指導	身體清潔護理									
	留置_____管路照護及注意事項									
	氧氣／抽痰使用方法及注意事項									
	傷口／造口之照護方式									
	衛教手冊提供：_____									
	定時返診追蹤的重要性									
	其他									
	衛教者簽名									
	病人或家屬簽名									

八、臨床路徑(Clinical Pathway)

1. **臨床路徑的發展緣由**：臨床路徑是為達提升醫療品質、監控醫療照護流程及控制醫療成本而產生的，是將醫療照護流程標準化，以確保大多數個案能在一定的醫療資源內，享有適當的醫療品質並達降低醫療成本之目的。

2. **臨床路徑的定義及效益**：執行臨床路徑在護理人員方面可作為照護指引、提高工作效率；在個案方面能獲得必要且適當的醫療處置與護理照護及衛生教育，減少住院天數、降低合併症及不必要的檢查；在醫院方面因個案住院天數減少進而提升病房使用率、降低醫療成本。故施行臨床路徑有三大好處：提升醫療品質、增進個案安全、減少醫療資源浪費。

3. **臨床路徑的內容**：其內容包括：檢查、檢驗、治療、藥物處置、飲食、護理照護、衛生教育、會診、出院計畫、預期住院天數及差異記錄。

4. **臨床路徑的施行步驟**：臨床路徑是根據某種特定的手術或診斷，由全體共同參與醫療照護的成員一同制定完成「醫療照護標準化流程」，以確保特定手術或診斷的個案能享有標準化的醫療照護，而達適當的醫療品質，雖然臨床路徑已將醫療照護流程標準化，但在執行臨床路徑時，仍需要注意到每位個案的個別性，以提供最適切的醫療照護。

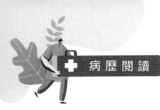

5. 臨床路徑範例

痔瘡切除術(Hemorrhoidectomy)　臨床路徑(P.1)

姓名		病歷號碼		床號		性別	□男 □女	科別	

	入院第一天(Pre-OP day)＿＿年＿＿月＿＿日 入院時間：＿＿＿＿＿	大夜	白班	小夜	入院第二天(OP day)＿＿年＿＿月＿＿日 Set to OR 時間：＿＿＿ 返回病房時間：＿＿＿	大夜	白班	小夜
麻醉					□半身 □全身 □IVG □其他：＿＿＿＿＿＿＿＿＿			
評估	□V/S：on ward routin 出血：量（1.多　2.中　3.少） 　　　顏色（1.鮮紅　2.暗紅　3.淡紅）	□ □	□ □	□ □	□術前：V/S：on ward routin □術後：V/S st.× 1 and q1h × 2 　　　Then on ward routine 　　　出血：量（1.多　2.中　3.少） 　　　　　顏色（1.鮮紅　2.暗紅　3.淡紅）	□ □	□ □	□ □
檢查	□CBC, PT, PTT, BS, BUN, Cr., GOT, GPT, Na, K, Cl □CXR：＿＿＿＿＿＿＿ ,□EKG：＿＿＿＿＿				異常 data：			
血品	備血：□PRBC：＿＿＿＿U □FFP：＿＿＿＿U 　　　□其他：＿＿＿＿＿＿＿U				輸血：□PRBC：＿＿＿＿U □FFP：＿＿＿＿U 　　　□其他：＿＿＿＿＿＿			
IV	Set IV. Cath：＿＿＿＿號；注射部位：＿＿＿＿				Set IV. Cath：＿＿＿＿號；注射部位：＿＿＿＿			
治療					□坐浴：＿＿＿＿＿次／天 □換藥：＿＿＿＿＿次／天	□ □	□ □	□ □
飲食	□NPO：時間＿＿＿＿ □低渣飲食 □水分攝取（至少 2,000c.c.~2,500c.c.／天）				□術前：NPO □術後：進食時間＿＿＿＿＿，採漸進式飲食			
活動	□無限制				□術前：無限制 □術後：第一次下床需有人陪伴			
排泄	排便：□無 □有 軟便劑：□PO □supp.				排便：術前：□無 □有 術後：□無 □有 術後解尿：□自解 at＿＿＿＿ □6hs.未解 □單導 at＿＿ ＿＿＿ c.c. □on foley at＿＿＿			
護理活動	□填寫麻醉同意書 □填寫手術同意書 □告 NPO □戴手圈 □確認手術部位已做標記 □傾聽、給予心理支持，減少手術壓力及恐懼				術前：□續 NPO 中 　　　□完成術前準備 □完成術前病患確認 術後：肛紗／□無 □有（移除肛紗 at＿＿＿＿） 　　　肛管／□無 □有（移除肛管 at＿＿＿＿） 　　　□傾聽、給予心理支持，協助疼痛處理			
疼痛	疼痛指數：(1~10 分)，□可忍受 □無法忍受 處理：□□服止痛藥可緩解 □打止痛針可緩解	□	□	□	疼痛指數：(1~10 分)，□可忍受 □無法忍受 處理：□□服止痛藥可緩解 □打止痛針可緩解	□	□	□
	經處理後疼痛指數：(1~10 分)	□	□	□	經處理後疼痛指數：(1~10 分)	□	□	□
衛教	□術前準備　　□術後照護 □水分攝取至少 2,000c.c.~2,500c.c.／天 □了解痔瘡切除的住院療程及預計出院日期				□溫水坐浴，＿＿＿＿次／天 & prn. □疼痛處理方式 □了解痔瘡切除的住院療程 □痔瘡切除術後照護			
其他特殊記錄								
簽名								

1.已執行以「ˇ」表示。　　2.個案了解衛教內容及已達目標以「△」表示。
3.不需要以「×」表示。　　4.需特別記錄以「※」表示。

痔瘡切除術(Hemorrhoidectomy)　臨床路徑(P.2)

姓名		病歷號碼		床號		性別	□男 □女	科別	

	入院第三天(POD 1)　___年___月___日	大夜	白班	小夜	入院第四天(POD 1)　___年___月___日	大夜	白班	小夜
評估	□V/S：on ward routin 傷口評估：出血量（1.多　2.中　3.少） 　　　　　顏色（1.鮮紅　2.暗紅　3.淡紅） 　　　　　血塊（1.多　2.中　3.少　4.無）	□ □ □	□ □ □	□ □ □	□V/S：on ward routin 傷口評估：出血量（1.多　2.中　3.少） 　　　　　顏色（1.鮮紅　2.暗紅　3.淡紅） 　　　　　血塊（1.多　2.中　3.少　4.無）	□ □ □	□ □ □	□ □ □
檢查	□輸血後 CBC/Hb._____ gm/dl							
血品	輸血：□PRBC：_____U □FFP：_____U 　　　□其他：_____U							
IV	□IV. Cath 留置 □注射部位外觀：_____				□Remove IV. Cath			
治療	□坐浴：_____次 □換藥：_____次				□坐浴：_____次 □換藥：_____次			
飲食	□溫和、高渣飲食 □水分攝取（至少 2,000c.c.~2,500c.c.／天）				□溫和、高渣飲食 □水分攝取（至少 2,000c.c.~2,500c.c.／天）			
活動	□無限制				□無限制			
排泄	排　便：□無 □有 □高纖飲食 軟便劑：□PO □supp.				排　便：□無　□有 □高纖飲食 軟便劑：□PO　□supp. 尿　液：□自解 □foley 留置			
護理活動	術後：肛紗／□無 □有（移除肛紗 at_____） 　　　肛管／□無 □有（移除肛管 at_____） 　　　□傾聽、給予心理支持，協助疼痛處理				□預約回診時間：___年___月___日，上、下午 診，_____號			
疼痛	疼痛指數：（1~10 分），□可忍受 □無法忍受 處理：□口服止痛藥可緩解 □打止痛針可緩解	□	□	□	疼痛指數：（1~10 分），□可忍受 □無法忍受 處理：□口服止痛藥可緩解 □打止痛針可緩解	□	□	□
	經處理後疼痛指數：（1~10 分）	□	□	□	經處理後疼痛指數：（1~10 分）	□	□	□
衛教	□傷口自我照顧情形 □溫水坐浴，能正確回示教 □溫和、高渣飲食 開立診斷書：（甲診：____份、乙診：____份）				出院衛教：□傷口自我照護　　□溫水坐浴 　　　　　□溫和、高渣飲食 □藥物使用 　　　　　□日常活動 □返診的重要性 開立診斷書：（甲診：____份、乙診：____份）			
其他特殊記錄								
簽名								

1.已執行以「ˇ」表示。　　2.個案了解衛教內容及已達目標以「△」表示。

3.不需要以「×」表示。　　4.需特別記錄以「※」表示。

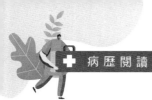

九、護理人員常用其他表單

生 命 徵 象 記 錄 表 (Vital Signs)

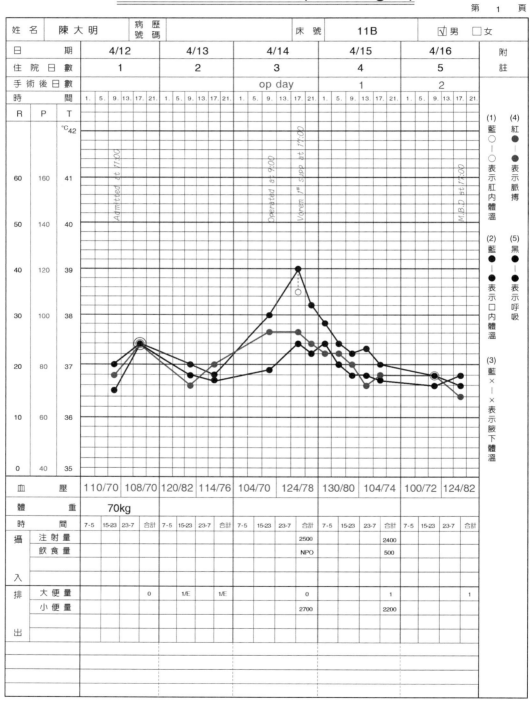

攝入／排出記錄表

姓　名				病 歷 號 碼				床　號		記 錄 日 期		年　月　日	
時	**攝**			**入**			**量**	**排**		**出**		**量**	
	注　　射　　量			飲		量	其　　他		尿　　量		大　　便	其　　他	
間				累計	種類	C.C gm	累計		累計	CC	累計	C.C/ 性質	累計		累計
8															
9															
10															
11															
12															
13															
14															
15															
小計															
16															
17															
18															
19															
20															
21															
22															
23															
小計															
24															
1															
2															
3															
4															
5															
6															
7															
小計															
總計															

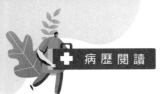
胰島素注射記錄表

第　頁

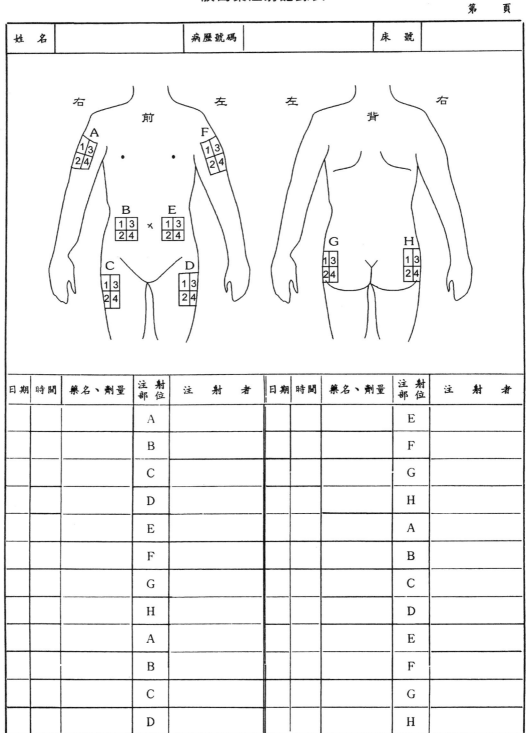

姓　名		病歷號碼		床　號	

日期	時間	藥名、劑量	注射部位	注　射　者	日期	時間	藥名、劑量	注射部位	注　射　者
			A					E	
			B					F	
			C					G	
			D					H	
			E					A	
			F					B	
			G					C	
			H					D	
			A					E	
			B					F	
			C					G	
			D					H	

給藥記錄單

姓　名：
病歷號：
床　號：
性　別：　　年齡：　　☐ 病患開刀

醫　師：　　科　別：
疾病名稱：
過敏記錄：
日　期：　　年　月　日　第　頁

類別	藥　品　說　明	用法、用量	本日給藥量	時間	給　藥　時　間　及　說　明												退藥量
					1	2	3	4	5	6	7	8	9	10	11	12	
				PM													
				AM													
			首日量：	尚存：	備註												
				PM													
				AM													
			首日量：	尚存：	備註												
				PM													
				AM													
			首日量：	尚存：	備註												
				PM													
				AM													
			首日量：	尚存：	備註												
				PM													
				AM													
			首日量：	尚存：	備註												
				PM													
				AM													
			首日量：	尚存：	備註												
				PM													
				AM													
			首日量：	尚存：	備註												
				PM													
				AM													
			首日量：	尚存：	備註												

類　別代　號	M—口服藥　　P—注射藥 S—水　藥　　E—外用藥	未　服　藥原因代號	△—檢查(NPO)　　　X—病患拒服 ○—病患不在　　　☆—暫停其他
藥師	給藥中班護士	給藥夜班護士	給藥早班護士　　　批價員

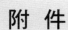

附 件

醫療機構施行手術及麻醉告知暨取得病人同意指導原則

2004 年 10 月 22 日公告

一、告知程序

（一）手術同意書與麻醉同意書一式兩份，由醫療機構人員先行完成「基本資料」之填寫。

（二）手術同意書部分，由手術負責醫師以中文填載「擬實施之手術」各欄，並依「醫師之聲明」1.之內容，逐項解釋本次手術相關資訊，同時於說明完成之各欄□內打勾。若手術負責醫師授權本次手術醫療團隊中之其他醫師，代為說明，手術負責醫師最後仍應確認已完全說明清楚，再將本同意書一份交付病人，如有其他手術或麻醉說明書，一併交付病人充分閱讀。麻醉同意書部分，由麻醉醫師以中文填載「擬實施之麻醉」各欄，依「醫師之聲明」1.之內容，逐項解釋本次手術麻醉相關資訊，同時於說明完成之各欄□內打勾。

（三）告知完成後，手術負責醫師、麻醉醫師應於相關同意書上簽名，並記載告知日期及時間。

（四）病人經過說明後，如有疑問，醫師應視手術之性質，給予合理充分的時間詢問及討論，並將病人問題記載於「醫師之聲明」2.，並加註日期及時間。

二、告知時應注意之事項

（一）應先了解病人對於醫療資訊接收之意願：

　　　對於醫療資訊之告知程度與方式，應尊重病人之意願，避免對其情緒及心理造成負面影響；告知前，應先探詢病人以了解病人接收醫療資訊之期望，如：(1)病人願意即時接受一切必要之醫療資訊；(2)僅需適時告知必要的醫療資訊；或(3)由醫師決定告知的內容等；(4)告知病人指定之人。

（二）告知之對象：

1. 以告知病人本人為原則。

2. 病人未明示反對時，亦得告知其配偶或親屬。

3. 病人為未成年人時，亦需告知其法定代理人。

4. 若病人意識不清或無決定能力，應告知其法定代理人、配偶、親屬或關係人。

5. 病人得以書面敘明僅向特定之人告知或對特定對象不予告知。

（三）如告知對象為病人之法定代理人、配偶、親屬或關係人時，不以當面告知之方式為限。

（四）醫師應盡可能滿足病人知悉病情及手術、麻醉資訊的需求，尊重病人自主權，以通俗易懂的辭彙及溫和的態度說明，避免誇大、威嚇之言語。

（五）醫療團隊其他人員亦應本於各該職業範疇及專長，善盡說明義務，盡可能幫助病人了解手術、麻醉過程中可能面臨的情況及應注意之事項等，對於病人或家屬所詢問之問題，如超越其專業範疇，應轉請手術負責醫師予以回答。

三、簽署手術同意書

（一）手術同意書除下列情形外，應由病人親自簽名：

1. 病人為未成年人或因故無法為同意之表示時，得由醫療法規定之人員（法定代理人、配偶、親屬或關係人）簽名。

2. 病人之關係人，原則上係指與病人有特別密切關係人，如同居人、摯友等；或依法令或契約關係，對病人負有保護義務之人，如監護人、少年保護官、學校教職員、肇事駕駛人、軍警消防人員等。

3. 病人不識字、亦無配偶、親屬或關係人可簽手術同意書時，得以按指印代替簽名，惟應有二名見證人。

（二）同意書之簽具，亦得請病人之親友為見證人，如病人無配偶、親屬可為見證人時，可請其關係人為之，證明病人已同意簽署同意書。

（三）醫療機構應於病人簽具手術同意書後一個月內，施行手術，逾期應重新簽具同意書，簽具手術同意書後病情發生變化者，亦同。

（四）醫療機構為病人施行手術後，如有再度為病人施行相同手術之必要者，仍應重新簽具同意書。

（五）醫療機構查核同意書簽具完整後，一份由醫療機構連同病歷保存，一份交由病人收執。

四、其他

（一）病人若病情危急，而病人之配偶、親屬或關係人不在場，亦無法取得病人本身之同意，需立即實施手術，否則將危及病人生命安全時，為搶救病人性命，依醫療法規定，得先為病人進行必要之處理。

（二）手術進行時，如發現建議手術項目或範圍有所變更，當病人之意識於清醒狀態下，仍應予告知，並獲得同意，如病人意識不清醒或無法表達其意思者，則應由病人之法定或指定代理人、配偶、親屬或關係人代為同意。無前揭人員在場時，手術負責醫師為謀求病人之最大利益，得依其專業判斷為病人決定之，惟不得違反病人明示或可得推知之意思。

（三）病人於簽具手術同意書後，仍得於手術前隨時主張拒絕施行手術治療，醫療機構得視需要，請病人於手術同意書載明並簽名。

（四）施行人工流產或結紮手術，應另依優生保健法之規定簽具手術同意書。

同意書

病人：_____　性別：_____　生日：_____年_____月_____日

病歷號碼：_____　床號：_____

因患_____

需實施_____

立同意書人經本院_____醫師（由醫師親自簽名）詳細說明下列事項：

　　需實行檢查（處置）之原因、注意事項及其必要性。

　　檢查（處置）成功率或可能發生之併發症及危險。

　　檢查（處置）給付：□健保　□自費　□部分自費。

　　並已充分了解上述事項，**□同意□不同意**由本院施行該項檢查（處置）。

　　本院實施檢查時，會善盡醫療上必要之注意事項以確保患者安全，過程中若發生緊急情況，同意接受本院必要之緊急處置。

　　此致

　　立同意書人：　　　　　　　簽章

　　身分證統一編號：

　　住址：

　　電話：

　　與病人之關係：

　　　　　　　　　　　　　　中華民國　　年　　月　　日

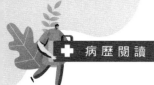

○○醫院（診所）手術同意書

＊基本資料

病人姓名_____

病人出生日期_____年_____月_____日

病人病歷號碼_____

手術負責醫師姓名_____

一、擬實施之手術（如醫學名詞不清楚，請加上簡要解釋）

1. 疾病名稱：

2. 建議手術名稱：

3. 建議手術原因：

二、醫師之聲明

1. 我已經盡量以病人所能了解之方式，解釋這項手術之相關資訊，特別是下列事項：

   □需實施手術之原因、手術步驟與範圍、手術之風險及成功率、輸血之可能性。

   □手術併發症及可能處理方式。

   □不實施手術可能之後果及其他可替代之治療方式。

   □預期手術後，可能出現之暫時或永久症狀。

   □如另有手術相關說明資料，我並已交付病人。

2. 我已經給予病人充足時間，詢問下列有關本次手術的問題，並給予答覆：

    (1) _____

    (2) _____

    (3) _____

手術負責醫師簽名：   日期：   年   月   日

                                          時間：   時   分

三、病人之聲明

1. 醫師已向我解釋，並且我已經了解施行這個手術的必要性、步驟、風險、成功率之相關資訊。

2. 醫師已向我解釋，並且我已經了解選擇其他治療方式之風險。

3. 醫師已向我解釋，並且我已經了解手術可能預後情況和不進行手術的風險。

4. 我了解這個手術必要時可能會輸血；我□同意 □不同意 輸血。

5. 針對我的情況、手術之進行、治療方式等，我能夠向醫師提出問題和疑慮，並已獲得說明。

6. 我了解在手術過程中，如果因治療之必要而切除器官或組織，醫院可能會將它們保留一段時間進行檢查報告，並且在之後會謹慎依法處理。

7. 我了解這個手術可能是目前最適當的選擇，但是這個手術無法保證一定能改善病情。

基於上述聲明，我同意進行此手術。

立同意書人簽名：   關係：病人之_____

住址：   電話：

日期：   年   月   日   時間：   時   分

見證人：   簽名：

日期：   年   月   日   時間：   時   分

附註：

一、一般手術的風險

1. 除局部麻醉以外之手術，肺臟可能會有一小部分塌陷失去功能，以致增加胸腔感染的機率，此時可能需要抗生素和呼吸治療。

2. 除局部麻醉以外之手術，腿部可能產生血管栓塞，並伴隨疼痛和腫脹。凝結之血塊可能會分散並進入肺臟，造成致命的危險，惟此種情況並不常見。

3. 因心臟承受壓力，可能造成心臟病發作，也可能造成中風。

4. 醫療機構與醫事人員會盡力為病人進行治療和手術，但是手術並非必然成功，仍可能發生意外，甚至因而造成死亡。

二、立同意書人非病人本人者，「與病人之關係欄」應予填載與病人之關係。

三、見證人部分，如無見證人得免填載。

○○醫院（診所）麻醉同意書

```
＊基本資料
病人姓名_____

病人出生日期_____年_____月_____日

病人病歷號碼_____

麻醉醫師姓名_____
```

一、擬實施之麻醉（如醫學名詞不清楚，請加上簡要解釋）

1. 外科醫師施行手術名稱：

2. 建議麻醉方式：

二、醫師之聲明

1. 我已經為病人完成術前麻醉評估之工作。

2. 我已經盡量以病人所能了解之方式，解釋麻醉之相關資訊，特別是下列事項：
   □麻醉之步驟。
   □麻醉之風險。
   □麻醉後，可能出現之症狀。
   □如另有麻醉相關說明資料，我並已交付病人。

3. 我已經給予病人充足時間，詢問下列有關本次手術涉及之麻醉問題，並給予答覆：
   (1) _____
   (2) _____
   (3) _____

麻醉醫師簽名：　　　　　　　　　　　　日期：　　年　　月　　日

　　　　　　　　　　　　　　　　　　　時間：　　時　　分

三、病人之聲明

1. 我了解為順利進行手術，我必須同時接受麻醉，以解除手術所造成之痛苦及恐懼。

2. 麻醉醫師已向我解釋，並且我已了解施行麻醉之方式及風險。

3. 我已了解附註之麻醉說明書。

4. 針對麻醉之進行，我能夠向醫師提出問題和疑慮，並已獲得說明。

　　基於上述聲明，我同意進行麻醉。

立同意書人簽名：　　　　　　　　　　　　關係：病人之_____
住址：　　　　　　　　　　　　　　　　　電話：
日期：　　年　　月　　日　　　　　　　　時間：　　時　　分

見證人：　　　　　　　　　　　　　　　　簽名：
日期：　　年　　月　　日　　　　　　　　時間：　　時　　分

附註：麻醉說明書

一、　由於您的病情，手術是必要的治療，而因為手術，您必須同時接受麻醉，除輔助手術順利施行外，可以使您免除手術時的痛苦和恐懼，並維護您生理功能之穩定，但對於部分接受麻醉之病人而言，或全身麻醉，或區域麻醉，均有可能發生以下之副作用及併發症：

1. 對於已有或潛在性心臟血管系統疾病之病人而言，於手術中或麻醉後較易引起突發性急性心肌梗塞。

2. 對於已有或潛在性心臟血管系統或腦血管系統疾病之病人而言，於手術中或麻醉後較易發生腦中風。

3. 緊急手術，或隱瞞進食，或因腹內壓高（如腸阻塞、懷孕等）之病人，於執行麻醉時有可能導致嘔吐，因而造成吸入性肺炎。

4. 對於特異體質之病人，麻醉可引發惡性發燒（這是一種潛在遺傳疾病，現代醫學尚無適當之事前試驗）。

5. 由於藥物特異過敏或因輸血而引致之突發性反應。

6. 區域麻醉有可能導致短期或長期之神經傷害。

7. 其他偶發之病變。

二、立同意書人非病人本人者，「與病人之關係欄」應予填載與病人之關係。

三、見證人部分，如無見證人得免填載。

學習評量

( )1. 有關護理記錄書寫的敘述下列何者為非？(A)護理記錄應具時效性　(B)護理記錄應越詳細越佳，所以要用很多的形容詞　(C)護理記錄應具體且量化為佳　(D)護理記錄應具組織性

( )2. 記錄在醫療照護上極為重要，其最主要目的在於？(A)教學參考　(B)評估　(C)提供溝通　(D)法律證明文件

( )3. 有關護理病歷的敘述下列何者為非？(A)了解主要入院因素　(B)進行收集個案基本資料　(C)進行初步護理評估　(D)記錄時機：於個案出院時使用

( )4. 有關手術前醫囑與護理記錄的敘述下列何者為非？(A)確認手術前應進行的各項醫囑　(B)確認手術前應進行的各項護理措施　(C)確認手術前應繳的醫療費用是否繳清　(D)確認手術前應進行的各項衛教

( )5. 有關出院護理摘要記錄的敘述下列何者為真？(A)於個案出院時作為目前病況摘要說明　(B)不需並列出出院時仍需持續進行的護理照護問題　(C)不需並列出院時各種管路　(D)不需並列出院時各項需衛教之內容

( )6. 下列何者不是施行臨床路徑的好處？(A)提升醫療品質　(B)減少護理工作量　(C)增進病人安全　(D)減少醫療資源浪費

( )7. 手術前需確認的事項下列何者為真？(A)個案身分　(B)手術方式及名稱　(C)個案身上標示的手術部位與病歷是否符合　(D)以上皆是

( )8. 手術前病患識別地點下列何者為非？(A)手術室內　(B)手術等待區　(C)恢復室內　(D)病患所屬單位（門診、病房、急診或加護病房）

( )9. 有關「護理衛教指導表」的敘述下列何者為非？(A)能依此表單進行有規劃、有系統地進行護理指導與衛教　(B)能依此表單清楚了解護理指導與衛教進行的進度　(C)能依此表單已執行護理指導與衛教的事項進行評值　(D)有進行護理指導與衛教一定要確實記錄於護理衛教指導表中，若有特殊事項不需書寫於護理記錄中

(　　)10. 執行臨床路徑在護理人員方面的助益，下列何者為非？(A)照護指引　(B)提高工作效率　(C)減少住院天數　(D)提供適當的衛生教育

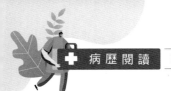
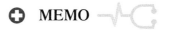

MEMO

14 | CHAPTER

電子病歷

作者｜林鳳映、陳麗琴、陳麗貞

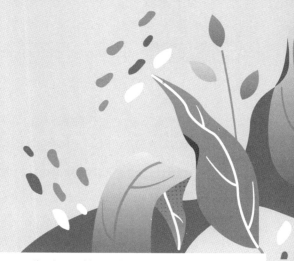

☑ 閱讀導引

1. 了解傳統紙本病歷與電子病歷的差異。
2. 了解電子病歷含括的內容。
3. 了解電子病歷交換平台系統架構。
4. 了解電子病歷發展歷程。
5. 了解電子病歷臨床實務應用。

　　病歷(Chart)是一種病人的醫學病史及醫療團隊人員照護過程的記錄。提供醫療團隊的溝通工具，以及法律上「書證」的文件記錄。由於電子時代的來臨，HIS 系統(Health Information System, HIS)醫療資訊的可近性及便利性，透過個人使用權限管理機制，提供介面輸入「密碼」及「代號」，就可查閱需要的病人相關病歷記錄及報告系統等資訊。

　　如此一來，簡化病歷人工調閱、傳送，同時不需耗時列印紙本存檔，重要的是提供及時性且正確性之病人醫療資訊，可以提高工作效率、減少資源浪費、降低醫療誤診、爭取醫療黃金期、提高醫療品質，且縮短了時空距離。於是衍生出「電子醫療記錄(Electronic Medical Records, EMR)」即「電子病歷」，取代傳統的「紙本病歷」。

14-1　電子病歷的範疇

　　儘管病歷型式由紙本轉為電子化，但應包含的項目必須完全相同。如：

1. 病人基本資料：包括姓名、電話、住址、緊急連絡人、語言、宗教信仰、種族、職業及保險公司種類等。

2. 病人主訴、過去病史及門診、急診、檢查治療診之相關醫療記錄，包括處方用藥史（藥名劑量、服用法、使用期限）、過敏史、手術史、診療記錄、懷孕史、接種疫苗歷程等。

3. 醫師檢查、理學檢查、手術及植入物記錄等。

4. 實驗室檢驗及診斷性檢查報告系統：包括放射線科檢查（X 光、電腦斷層掃描）、微生物檢驗（血液培養）、其他特殊檢查（切片）等。

5. 診療計畫：住院診療及出院計畫，化學療法藥物種類及用法，或放射線物理治療、心理諮商等。

6. 每日病程記錄：住院期間病情變化、會診、處置及治療，疼痛、營養、復健等評估後續追蹤。

7. 護理記錄：護理過程包含：評估、計畫、措施、評值及病人家屬衛教指導等後續追蹤。

8. 其他醫事人員記錄：醫事人員執行記錄包含：營養師、復健師、心理師、社工師呼吸治療師等。

紙本病歷與電子病歷的比較詳見表 14-1。

表 14-1　紙本病歷與電子病歷的比較

比較項目	紙本病歷	電子病歷
執行面	手寫費時、字跡潦草、不易辨讀	鍵打，省時省力、字體清晰、一目了然
查詢面	資料查詢不易，需一頁頁翻查	軟體設計分類精細，「按鍵」即刻顯現，且可以圖表方式表示，易於解讀
環保面	紙張材料不環保，資料易失落且不易儲存，較占空間	電子庫的存量大，而且可以永久儲存，不占空間
設備面	單純、簡易，不怕當機，維護費低	若電腦當機，則運作全部停止。設備及維修費高，需經專業訓練才會操作
資料面	記錄不易修改，且留痕跡	修改簡易，保留增刪及補述記錄可循
隱私性	取得不易，非本院所醫療人員，無法取得病人資料	暴露性高，需設置「防護牆」，加上醫療院所及團隊人員私密金鑰（具有配對關係之數位資料）或驗證數位簽章者
問題提示	靠人工判讀，如無知識及經驗，可能無法得知問題之所在	軟體設計，即可提出「警訊」，或系統自動啟動管控機制
診治建議	靠人工尋找會診記錄較零散	由軟體設計會顯示出尚缺何種檢查或藥物使用或治療等建議
資訊改正	無法告知填錯欄位或誤寫	軟體設計可管控「人為」疏失機制
責任歸屬	筆跡鑑定	靠特定「電子簽章」，權限「代號」或「密碼」
用藥記錄	逐字手寫，字體不一、拼錯字、誤讀機會大，藥與藥之間的互相影響及副作用無法顯示	字體清晰，同時會提示藥的副作用及相互抵制的警語、意見。尤其用量途徑的說明，以達到「零」錯誤

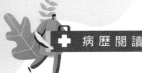
表 14-1　紙本病歷與電子病歷的比較（續）

比較項目	紙本病歷	電子病歷
複製	1. 必須一頁頁翻找，費時又費力 2. 不易察覺資料不完整或遺失	軟體會自動彙整結果及歸類整理，如： 1. 實驗室報告以最近「三個月」為先 2. 用藥記錄以「一年」為期限 3. 住院記錄以「最近 10 次」為準 4. 手術記錄則全部保留 5. 病人主訴，依時序列出，以最近兩年為主 6. 診斷則依症狀、時序列出，且有代碼顯示，屬於「active」或「inactive」，且依序由頭／頸／心／肺／腹／四肢／神經系統／一般或其他領域逐一列出
整合度	單向且單一記錄無法整合	能與百科全書或實證文獻多面向連結，輔助臨床問題之解決，提升醫療品質，降低醫療失誤，減少資源浪費
評估面	由許多單位分別評估再人工整理	透過系統整理、分類，即可得到評估整合結果之數據及資料
同意書效力	「手術同意書」紙本當事人親自簽署具法律效力	目前軟體系統尚無法取得自然人憑證之法律效力，無法取代當事人親自簽署效力，可透過紙本與 PDF 檔案同時保存

14-2　電子病歷相關規範

　　衛生福利部於 2000 年著手研擬「電子病歷交換與整合機制」，歷經十年，電子簽章法施行細則於 2002 年 4 月 10 日發布，公告實施病歷電子化，且設立「中央資料庫」備有「索引」，達到全國病歷透明化，意即每家醫療院所可藉由「中央資料庫」蒐取需要的「個案病歷」。

指令：必須符合臨床文件標準架構(Clinical Document Architecture Release Two, CDA R2)制訂的 HL 7 (Health Level 7)引用範例為準則，如此我國將來才易與國際醫療接軌。

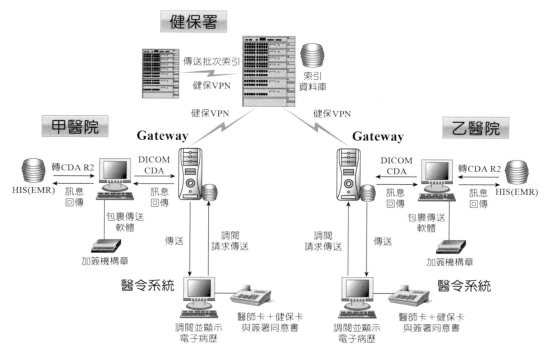

1. VPN：Virtual Private Network，全國醫療影像交換中心網站交換系統代號辨識。

2. Gateway：閘道器（各個醫院內 EMR 資料蒐集中心）。

3. DICOM：Digital Imagine and Communication in Medicine，醫療文字交換以 Health Level 7(HL7)為準，醫療影像交換以影像 DICOM 為準。

4. CDA：Clinical Documentation Architecture，臨床文件標準架構，使申報的臨床文件報告，有一致性的標準，全球性通用。

5. HIS：Health Information System，健康資訊系統。

圖 14-1　電子病歷交換平台系統架構圖

參考資料：衛生福利部電子病歷推動專區 http://emr.mohw.gov.tw/news.aspx。

其中閘道器(Gateway)即為各家醫療院所內的電子病歷資料蒐集中心，衛生福利部將要交換的電子病歷依「VPN」（索引）轉送到「電子病歷交換中心」儲存，日後其他醫療院所使用自有的「醫令系統」（整合交換系統）或登入「電子

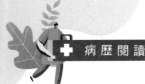
病歷交換中心」的「web」（網站）擷取 VPN（索引），則可瀏覽 EMR。以下簡述衛生福利部公布的「血液檢驗報告交換內容基本格式」（表 14-2）。

表 14-2　血液檢驗報告交換內容基本格式

項次	區塊描述	欄位名稱	LOINC[1]	欄位說明
1	醫療機構代碼	醫療機構代碼 Hospital ID		[1..1][2]
2	醫療機構名稱	醫療機構名稱 Hospital Name		[1..1]
3	病人基本資料	身分證字號 ID Number		[1..1] 身分證號 護照號碼 居留證號
4		病歷號碼 Chart Number		[1..1]
5		姓名 Name		[1..1]
6		性別 Gender		[1..1]
7		出生日期 Birth Date		[1..1]
8	檢驗單號	檢驗單號 Application No.		[1..1]院所系統之號碼
9	檢體來源	檢體來源 Sampling Source		[1..1]如肝、某靜脈…
10	檢體類別	檢體類別 Categories		[1..1]如血液、尿
11	檢體類別說明	檢體類別 Categories Description		[1..1]如血液、尿
12	檢體項目代號	健保檢驗項目代號 Test Item Code		[1..1]如 0800IC
13	檢驗項目名稱	健保檢驗項目名稱 Test Item Name		[1..1]如紅血球計數

表 14-2　血液檢驗報告交換內容基本格式（續）

項次	區塊描述	欄位名稱	LOINC[1]	欄位說明
14	採檢日期、時間	採檢日期、時間 Sampling Date & Time		[1..1]
15	收件日期、時間	收件日期、時間 Delivering Date and Time		[0..1][3]
16	檢驗報告結果	檢驗報告結果 Testing Results	Relevant Diagnostic Test and/or Laboratory Data	[1..*]17~24 項次欄位內容可重覆出現
		項次 Item Number		[1..1]如 CBC 具有多個檢驗結果項次
17		報告日期、時間 Report Date and Time		[1..1]
18		檢驗項目名稱 LOINC Long Name		[1..1]LOINC
19		檢驗報告結果值 Value		[1..1]如 positive
20		單位 Units		[1..1]如 mg/mL
21		檢驗方法 Method		[0..1]如酵素免疫分析法 (EIA)
22		參考值 Reference		[1..]如 0~25
23		備註 Remark		[0..1]
24		醫事人員姓名 Technician Name		[1..*][4] 包括臨床醫師及檢驗技師

備註：

1. LOINC：Logical Observation Identifiers Name and Code，對應名稱。
2. [1..1]：此欄位為必選，且只有一次。
3. [0..1]：此欄位為可選，且只有一次。
4. [1..*]：此欄位為必選，可重覆出現。
5. [0..*]：此欄位為可選，可重覆出現。

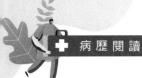

14-3　電子病歷的發展歷程

　　根據美國病歷協會的定義，病歷邁入完全電子化需經過五大歷程，分別為：

1. **醫療記錄自動化**(Automated Medical Records, AMR)：運用電腦化與資訊化列印代替手寫病歷，醫療記錄自動將檢驗資料及病人條碼刷入系統，透過機器直接傳送到「醫令系統」儲存，取代昔日以書面複製貼上的作法。

2. **醫療記錄電腦化**(Computerized Medical Records, CMR)：病歷資料運用數位多媒體儲存，此歷程中是「影像資料電腦化」，如 X 光片、電腦斷層掃描、攝影等（EKG 除外），取代「實片」的傳閱，節省儲存空間及避免遺失，國內已有多家大型醫療院所實施。

3. **電子醫療記錄**(Electronic Medical Records, EMR)：經由電子化資料庫路徑重組，以時序作數位化處理，可藉由網路傳輸提供資料共享介面，將病人資訊經由電腦「伺服器」加上「軟體」運作。以衛生福利部公布的「門診用藥格式與標準規範」做簡要說明（表 14-3）。

表 14-3　門診用藥交換內容基本格式欄位需求清單（2010.9.17 版本）

項次	區塊描述	欄位名稱	LOINC 對應名稱	欄位說明
1	醫療機構	醫療機構代碼 Hospital ID		[1..1]
2		醫療機構名稱 Hospital Name		[1..1]
3	病人 基本資料	身分證號 Personal ID No.		[1..1]身分證號、護照號碼或居留證號
4		病歷號碼 Chart No.		[1..1]
5		姓名 Name		[1..1]
6		性別 Gender		[1..1]
7		出生日期 Birth Date		[1..1]

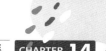

表 14-3　門診用藥交換內容基本格式欄位需求清單（2010.9.17 版本）（續）

項次	區塊描述	欄位名稱	LOINC 對應名稱	欄位說明
8	門診日期	門診日期 O.P.D. Date		[1..1]
9	科別	科別 Department		[1..1]
10	診斷	診斷 Diagnosis		[1..*]
11	處方箋 種類	處方箋種類註記 Types of Prescription	Medication prescribed	[1..1]，一般處方、慢性病連續處方箋等
12	藥品細項	項次 Item		[1..1]
13		藥品代碼 Drug Code		[1..1]
14		藥品商名稱 Brand Name		[1..1]
15		學名 Genetic Name		[1..1]
16		劑型 Dosage Form		[1..1]如藥丸、藥水
17		劑量 Dose		[1..1]
18		劑量單位 Dose Unit		[1..1]如顆、c.c.
19		頻率 Frequency		[1..1]如 QW1 是每星期一使用；BIW 是每兩週使用 1 次；Q6H 是每 6 小時使用 1 次；QDHS 是每天睡前使用 1 次
20		給藥途徑 Route of Administration		[1..1]如 PO 為口服；IM 為肌肉注射；EXT 為外用
21		給藥日數 Medication Days		[1..1]

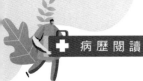

表 14-3　門診用藥交換內容基本格式欄位需求清單（2010.9.17 版本）（續）

項次	區塊描述	欄位名稱	LOINC 對應名稱	欄位說明
22	藥品細項	給藥總量 Total Amount		[1..1]
23		給藥總單位 Total Units		[1..1]如顆、瓶、c.c.
24		實際給藥總量 Actual Amount		[1..1]
25		實際給藥總單位 Actual Units		[1..1]如顆、瓶、c.c.
26		磨粉註記 Powdered		[1..1] 應磨粉「Y」 不應磨粉「N」
27		註記說明 Note		[0..1]空白欄位用於註記說明
28	醫師姓名	醫師姓名 Physician Name		[1..1]

　　美國、歐洲、澳洲之國際標準化組織如：ASTM、HL 7 與 HIMSS 建立電子病歷標準，採用以開放性原始碼的電子病歷導入。目前國內許多教學醫院及醫療機構開始實施「門診用藥」、「檢（驗）查報告」等之電子病歷。然而部分醫院如長庚紀念醫院已於 2010 年 1 月參與衛生福利部委託研究計畫，成立「電子病歷推動委員會」運作組織架構，陸續進行全國性體系內機構及全面化「病歷記錄」及「護理記錄」之電子簽章，同時報備衛生福利部及公告實施電子簽章項目不列印紙本作業。硬體設備評估包含：建置電子簽章無線網域之可近性環境，安裝 E 化工作行動電腦及讀卡機等周邊設備，結合病人照護流程，於記錄同時以衛生福利部核發的「醫事人員卡」插入推車上的讀卡機，HIS 系統輸入使用者名稱及密碼，自動驗證各職務人員可使用權限後，即可登入「醫囑系統」或「護理資訊系統」，執行醫療或護理照護記錄及簽章作業，包含：診療記錄、醫囑執行治療記錄、醫囑用藥與護理給藥作業之一藥一簽記錄、護理過程、手術準備及護理記錄等。

4. **電子病人資訊**(Electronic Patient Records, EPR)：院際間整合平台及基本醫療記錄流通，所有病人的病情評估、醫囑用藥、臨床處置等全面推展「行動化電子病歷」及「無紙化」。至 2019 年 5 月已有 404 家醫療院所完成建置。

5. **電子健康資訊**(Electronic Health Records, EHR)：廣泛性應用病人健康資料，所有醫療機構的資訊，可以透過「網站」或「資訊中心」傳遞，完全透明化，達到資訊共享的境界。

　　依據衛生福利部統計資料指出，目前國內有近七成的醫療院所可提供電子病歷交換，除了醫院內資訊系統與資料庫的整合外，院際間合作及資料交換應用的目標也逐漸達成，也就是說「以病人為中心」的理念將來可以病人病歷資訊跟著病人走。電子病歷發展過程當然更需要衛生福利部由法規面、執行面、標準面、安全面，適時增（修）訂相關法規，以提供醫院機構執行及推展電子病歷之依循。

14-4　電子病歷的實務應用

　　電子病歷實施應訂有操作人員與系統建置、維護、稽核、管制之標準作業程序，並有執行記錄可供查核，電子病歷之簽名或蓋章，應以電子簽章方式為之，應於病歷製作後 24 小時內完成之。於臨床實務應用應確實符合醫療法規相關規定，同時掌握實施過程應注意事項，如：(1)電子病歷之製作、記錄刪改及儲存須符合醫療法第 68~70 條之規定，應予保留；(2)病歷資訊系統建置，應具備完善之標準作業程序、明確規範使用者權限及查核管控機制；(3)電子病歷使用記錄應併同電子病歷保存，且有備源及緊急應變辦法；(4)必須有資訊安全防護系統，以確保電子病歷之安全性及隱私性維護；(5)資訊系統所製作之電子病歷資料，電子簽章應憑中央主管機關核發之醫事憑證為之。須使用醫事憑證簽章，並經中央主管機關加註時戳，以確認電子病歷之不可否認性；(6)病歷保存期間內，電子病歷之存取、增刪、查閱、複製等事項，及其執行人員、時間及內容保有完整記錄，可供查核。

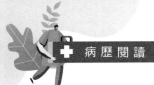

　　以長庚紀念醫院實施及推展經驗，依電子病歷推行委員會為中心統籌電子病歷實施計畫時程，建立作業準則與標準作業程序，確實執行緊急應變人員教育訓練及演練，以及推動電子病歷資訊院際間互通作業，定期彙整實施成效並檢討改善。

　　以下將以護理作業系統之護理記錄電子簽章執行流程為例說明醫囑下達到護理人員處理醫囑的流程：

　　醫師開立醫囑後，護理人員於線上核對後執行醫囑，並將相關照護處置執行撰寫護理記錄。撰寫護理記錄後需先輸入預簽章護理記錄內容之起迄時間，在電腦讀卡機上插入醫事人員卡，輸入個人醫事人員卡密碼，電腦驗證無誤後執行電子簽章，簽章成功或失敗會於簽章訊息欄中呈現。最後於下班前檢視記錄之正確及完整性後列印出來並製作成書面病歷。

　　以下為護理人員製作病歷模擬畫面及電子簽章相關設備。

一、護理資訊系統之操作模擬畫面

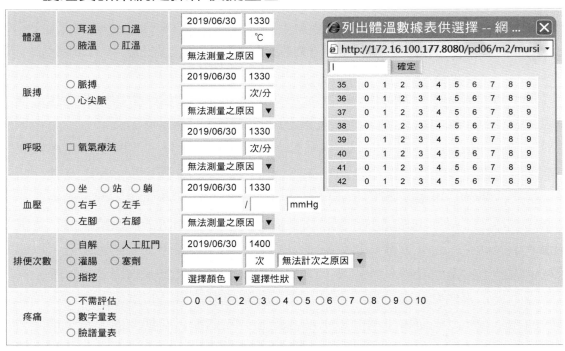

圖 14-2　生命徵象記錄表輸入模擬畫面

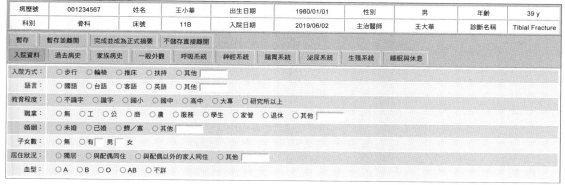

圖 14-3　護理評估表表輸入模擬畫面

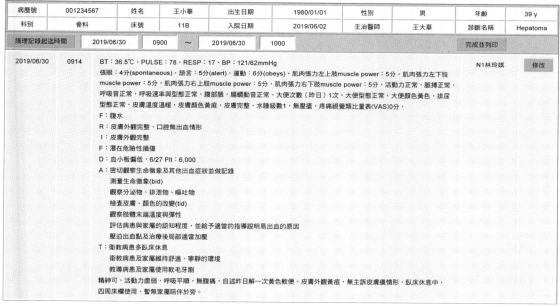

圖 14-4　護理記錄表輸入模擬畫面

實際操作步驟：

→打開護理作業—NIS 系統—護理記錄電子簽章資訊化畫面

→確認醫事卡之基本資料成功

→Pin 碼驗證成功

→使用一般型讀卡機

→驗驗中

→上傳電子病歷資料庫成功

簽章結束後，頁尾自動產生註記符號，如：⊕電子簽章

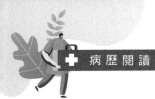

二、電子簽章相關設備：包括讀卡機、醫事人員卡

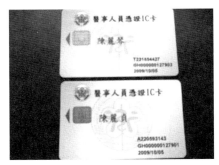

圖 14-5　醫事人員卡

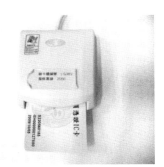 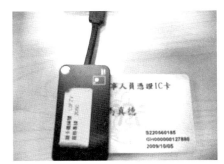

圖 14-6　讀卡機插入醫事人員卡

結　論

　　科技的發達致使駭客成為「隱私權」是一大挑戰。另涉及「醫療糾紛」的審核依據，電子病歷的誠信度也受到威脅。依據現行公告「電子簽章法令規範」實務執行時，應訂定醫療機構規章制度且確實監控管理病人資料安全，包含操作人員與系統建置、維護、稽核、管制之標準作業程序，並有執行記錄可供查核，以防止「原始記錄被竄改」，甚至造成嚴重後果不堪設想。醫療資訊持續發展及建置 HIS 系統完整性，提供跨領域醫療團隊間資訊連結功能與流通，而且是「無紙化」、「透明化」、「安全化」、「普及化」。

 掃描　 醫療機構電子病歷製作及管理辦法　 電子簽章法

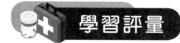 **學習評量**

1. 目前所使用的電子病歷軟體中，有一項辦不到的是＿＿＿＿＿＿＿＿＿。

2. 電子病歷資訊交換標準：醫療文字以＿＿＿＿＿＿＿＿＿、醫療影像以 為標準。

3. 我國健保在＿＿＿＿＿年實施門診用藥病歷電子化。

4. 期待 10 年後國民的「健康史」能達到哪四化？
   ＿＿＿＿＿＿＿＿＿、＿＿＿＿＿＿＿＿＿、＿＿＿＿＿＿＿＿＿、＿＿＿＿＿＿＿＿＿。

5. EMR 全文是 Electronic ＿＿＿＿＿＿ Records。

6. EHR 全文是＿＿＿＿＿＿＿＿＿＿＿＿＿＿＿＿＿＿＿＿＿＿＿。

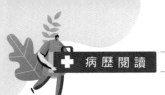
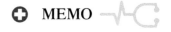
MEMO

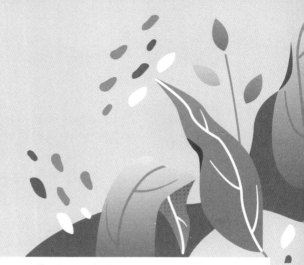

15 | CHAPTER

各科病歷範例

作者｜陳滄山、陳瑋芬、周志和
釋高上、郭彥志、王惠芳

☑ 閱讀導引

1. 認識神經內科病歷記錄內容。
2. 認識肝膽腸胃科病歷記錄內容。
3. 認識婦產科病歷記錄內容。
4. 認識新陳代謝科病歷記錄內容。
5. 認識骨科病歷記錄內容

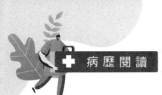

15-1 Neurology

Admission Note

Neurology service, 55 year-old male, married, merchant.

Date of admission: 2023-12-21.

Chief Complaint:

Acute onset of difficult swallowing since 2023/12/21 morning.

Present Illness:

The 55 year-old man denied any systemic disease before. He has suffered from acute onset of difficult swallowing since 12/21 morning after waking up. He couldn't eat anything including water and food since then. Besides, he also complained of mild numbness over his right face and left limbs. Mild slurred speech was also noted by his family. He denied diplopia, incoordination of limbs, or gait problems. Mild ptosis on the right side was told in the neurology clinic.

He was admitted under the impression of acute stroke.

Past History:

1. Denied any systemic disease or operation history.
2. No known food or drug allergy.

Personal History:

1. Habit of smoking: 0.5 pack per day for 3~4 years.
2. Habit of alcohol consumption: Social, 2~3 days per week recently, 4~5 bottles beer.
3. Habit of betel nut chewing: Denied.
4. The history of drug abuse: Denied.

Family History:

1. HTN: Mother, brothers.
2. Stroke: Mother.

Review of Systems:

1. Eyes: Loss of vision(-), distorted vision(-), floaters(-), eye pain(-), light sensitivity(-), double vision(-), redness(-), discharge(-), foreign body sensation(-), itching(-), excessive tearing(-).
2. Constitutional system: Fever(-), chills(-), weight loss(-), weight gain(+), fatigue(-), loss of appetite(-).
3. ENT: Hearing difficulty(-), vertigo(-), ear pain(-), ringing in ears(-), runny nose(-), post-nasal drip(-), nose bleeds(-), dry mouth(+), hoarseness(-), frequent sore throat(-).
4. Cardiovascular: Chest pain(-), palpitation(-), shortness of breath with exertion(+).
5. Respiratory: Cough(+), chronic shortness of breath(-), wheezing(-), coughing up blood(-).
6. GI: Swallowing difficulty(-), vomiting(-), diarrhea(-), constipation(-), change in appearance of stool(-), chronic abdominal pain(-), yellow skin(-).
7. GU: Urinary frequency(+), urinary pain(-), blood(-), discharge(-), mass(-).
8. Muscular-skeletal: Back pain(-), joint pain(-), joint swelling(-), joint redness(-), muscle pain(-), muscle cramp(-).
9. Skin: Skin rash(-), itching(-), chronic dry skin(-).
10. Neurological: Headache(-), numbness(+), weakness(-), fainting(-), slurred speech(+), seizures(-), tremor(-), dizziness(-).
11. Psychiatric: Anxiety(-), depression(-), memory loss(-), difficulty concentration(-), phobias(-).
12. Endocrine: Heat or cold intolerance(-), excessive thirst(+), excessive hunger(+), excessive urination(+).
13. Hematology/Immunology: Swollen lymph node(-).

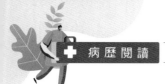
Physical Examination:

1. General appearance: Fair.

2. BW: 80 kg, BH: 170 cm.

3. Vital sign: BT: 36.7°C, PR: 72/min, RR: 18/min, BP: 182/120 mmHg.

4. HEENT: No anemic conjunctiva, anicteric sclera, no gum bleeding, no tonsillar enlargement, no throat erythematous.

5. Neck: Supple. No jugular vein engorgement, no palpable lymph node, normal sized thyroid gland. No carotid bruit.

6. Chest and lungs: Symmetric expansion. Resonance on percussion in all lung fields. Clear breath sound. No crackles, wheeze, or stridor.

7. Heart: Regular heart beats, no murmur.

8. Abdomen: Flat, normoactive bowel sound, no shifting dullness, no tenderness or rebound tenderness.

9. Extremities: Normal muscle power. No deformity, free joint movement.

10. Peripheral pulsations: Normal and equal in carotid, brachial, popliteal and dorsopedal arteries.

Neurologic Examination:

1. Consciousness: Clear and alert. Orientated to time, place and person.

2. Cranial nerve:
   (1) CN2: No visual field defect, prompt pupillary light reflex, pupillary size: R/L: 2 mm/3 mm.
   (2) CN3, 4, 6: Full range of motion. Right eye partial ptosis.
   (3) CN5: Decreased pinprick, light touch, and temperature sensation over right face. Masseter muscle: Symmetric and full muscle power.
   (4) CN7: No central facial palsy. Normal taste function.
   (5) CN8: No hearing impairment by finger rubbing.
   (6) CN9, 10: No uvular deviation. Gag reflex: +/+.
   (7) CN11: Muscle power of SCM and trapezius: Symmetric and full.
   (8) CN12: No tongue deviation.

3. Sensory function: Decreased pinprick, light touch, and temperature sensation in left limbs and body.

4. Motor function:

　　(1) Normal muscle power R/L: 5/5.

　　(2) DTR: Normal on both sides.

　　(3) Babinski sign R/L: -/-.

5. Coordination:

　　(1) FNF: Mild ataxia on right arm.

　　(2) HNS: Mild ataxia on right leg.

6. Bowel and bladder control: No fecal or urinary incontinence.

Laboratory:

1. CBC

Date	WBC	RBC	Hb	Hct	PLT	MCV	MCHC	MCH
2023/12/21	8,000/uL	5.42×10⁶/uL	17.5 g/dL	51%	250,000/uL	90 fL	30 g/dL	30 pg

2. Differential count

Date	Neutrophils	Lymphocytes	Monocytes	Eosinophils	Basophils
2023/12/21	75%	15%	6%	3%	0.1%

3. BCS

Date	Glucose (AC)	BUN	Creatinine	AST	ALT	Sodium	Potassium
2023/12/21	247 mg/dL	20 mg/dL	0.8 mg/dL	24 U/L	26 U/L	135 mEq/L	4.1 mEq/L
Date	Cholesterol	TG	LDL-C	HDL-C	UA	HbA$_{1c}$	–
2023/12/22	300 mg/dL	450 mg/dL	148 mg/dL	62 mg/dL	7.3 mg/dL	10.2%	–

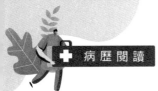

Neurological Localization:

Wallenberg syndrome, suspect acute stroke at the right side of the lateral medulla.

Impression:

Suspect brainstem stroke.

Diagnostic Plans:

Arrange brain image (brain CT and brain MRI).

Therapeutic Plans:

1. Adequate fluid hydration.
2. Survey the risk factors of stroke.
3. Check GCS and monitor blood sugar Q6H.

Educational Plans:

1. Cessation of smoking.
2. Exercise.

Attending Physician: ×××

Resident: △△△

Progress Notes

Neurology service, 55 year-old male, married, merchant.

Date of admission: 2023-12-21.

2023-12-22

#1 Suspect brainstem stroke

O:

1. Wallenberg syndrome, no deterioration of neurological signs.

2. Brain CT didn't show ICH or large cerebral infarcts.

A: Suspect brainstem infarct.

P:

1. Add antiplatelet (Aspirin).

2. Arrange brain MRI.

3. Stroke risk factors survey.

4. Consult physiatrist.

#2 Dyslipidemia

O: Hypercholesteremia.

A: Dyslipidemia.

P:

1. Add Statin.

2. Diet control and regular exercise.

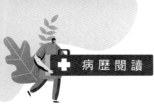

#3 hyperglycemia

O: HbA$_{1c}$=10.2%.

A: Diabetes mellitus type 2, poor control.

P:

> 1. Check finger stick blood sugar.
>
> 2. Insulin PRN usage.
>
> 3. Diet control and regular exercise.

Attending Physician: ××××

Resident: △△△

2023-12-23

#1 Suspect brainstem stroke

O:

> 1. Wallenberg syndrome.
>
> 2. Brain MRI showed acute infarction over right lateral posterior medullary area.

A: Right lateral posterior medullary infarct.

P:

> 1. Adequate fluid hydration.
>
> 2. Closely follow-up neurological signs.

Attending Physician: ×××

Resident: △△△

Order Sheet

Neurology service, 55 year-old male, married, merchant.

Date of admission: 2023-12-21.

Standing Order

2023-12-22

Diagnosis:

1. Wallenberg syndrome, suspect brainstem infarct.

2. Diabetes mellitus type 2.

3. Dyslipidemia.

Activity: Bed rest.

Allergies: No known food or drug allergy.

Take BP, PR, RR QID.

Take blood sugar QID.

Check GCS and muscle power QID.

Diet: On NG tube diet 1,750 Kcal.

Medications:

1. IVF: N/S run 60 mL/hr.

2. Trandate 1/2 amp IV push prn if SBP >220 mmHg or DBP >130 mmHg.

Attending Physician: ×××

Resident: △△△

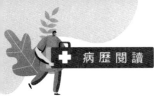

Stat Order

1. Insulin Actrapid 10U SC PRN (if BS>250).

2. Check glucose (fasting) × 1 stat.

3. Check BUN (blood urea nitrogen) × 1 stat.

4. Check CRP × 1 stat.

5. Check CBC-I (WBC, RBC, Hb, HCT, PLT) × 1 stat.

6. Check creatinine × 1 stat.

7. Check K (Potassium) × 1 stat.

8. Check Na (Sodium) × 1 stat.

9. Check WBC differential count × 1 stat.

10. Check chol, TG, HDL-C, LDL-C, HbA$_{1c}$ uric acid CM.

11. Arrange bran CT without contrast stat.

Attending Physician: × × ×

Resident: △△△

Radiology Reports

2023-12-22

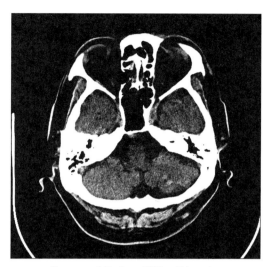

figure 15-1　CT of brain

CT of brain without contrast medium shows:

1. There is normal brain parenchymal configuration and gyration pattern.
   The basal ganglia and thalami are unremarkable.
   The gray white matter differentiation is intact.
2. There is no abnormal ventricular dilatation.
3. The skull bone shows no fracture lines.

Impression: Early infarction was not totally ruled out.

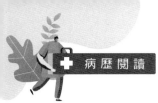

2023-12-23

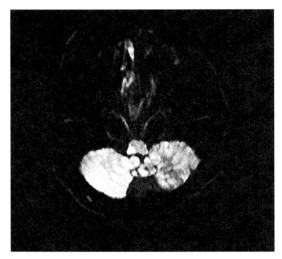

figure 15-2　MRI of brain

MRI of brain without contrast medium shows:

1. Presence of lesion involving right postolateral medulla oblongata with low SI on T1WI, and high SI on T2WI, flair, and DWI.

2. Presence of lesions involving right occipital periventricular white matter region with hypointense on T1WI, high SI on T2WI, and no high SI change on DWI.

3. Encephalomalacia change at the inferior part of L't cerebellum.

4. Presence of dilatation of all ventricles and proportional widening of bilateral cerebral sulci.

5. Nearly total occlusion of the distal part of right intradural vertebral artery.

6. Short segmental severe thrombotic stenosis of left intradural vertebral artery.

7. Paranasal sinusitis.

Impression: Acute infarction involving right postolateral medulla oblongata.

Consultation Sheet

姓名：○○○　　病歷號碼：××××××　床號：××　　　　出生日期：××××××

性別：男　　　入院日期：××××××　開單科別：神經內科　照會科別：復健科

The middle-aged male had acute right lateral-posterior medullary infarction. He presented severe dysarthria and dysphagia. NG tube feeding was placed on. Please arrange swallowing rehabilitation for him. Thank you.

Dr. ××× at 2023-12-22 4:00 p.m.

Reply Sheet

Dear Dr.×××,

The man with acute medullary infarction was evaluated. Swallowing vedio-esophagram and rehabilitation program will be arranged. Thank you.

Dr. ○○○ at 2023-12-23 10:30 a.m.

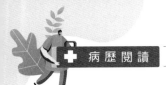

15-2 Hepatology and Gastroenterology

Admission Note

Hepatology and Gastroenterology, 54 years old, female, married, dormitory administrator.

Date of admission: 2023-1-12.

Chief Complaint:

Sudden-onset severe abdominal pain in RUQ for ten hours.

Present Illness:

This 54 year-old female patient suffered from a sudden-onset of abdominal pain at her RUQ for ten hours. The continuing colicky pain made her unable to walk. It also radiated to her right shoulder. It may be relieved by compression over her abdomen. She also felt nauseous, but there were no diarrhea, constipation, hematochezia, or jaundice. She then took some Acetaminophen and the pain only relieved for a moment. Four hours later, the pain intensified. She went to the health center in the next day and the doctor found gallstones by ultrasound. Then the doctor transferred her to our ER.

At the ER, her vital signs were stable. Physical examination showed remarkable Murphy's sign. Blood examination showed leukocytosis. Abdominal ultrasound revealed dilated common bile duct and thickening of the gallbladder wall. Acute cholecystitis was the diagnosis. She was admitted to receive antibiotic therapy.

Past History:

1. Systemic disease: AIDS(-), HBV(-), HCV(-), COPD(-), CVA(-), DM(-), HTN(+), hyperlipidemia(+).
2. Hospitalization: Denied.
3. Operation: Denied.

4. The history of drug abuse: Denied.

5. Habit of alcohol consumption: Denied.

6. Habit of smoking: Denied.

7. Habit of betel nut chewing: Denied.

8. Allergic history: Denied.

Family History:

Her father died of AMI at age 60. Her mother has hypertension. There are one elder brother and younger sister as her siblings. Her younger sister has asthma.

Physical Examination:

1. Consciousness: Clear and oriented.

2. HEENT:
   Eyes: Pinkish conjunctivae, anicteric sclera.
   Prompt and symmetric pupillary reflex.
   No grossly evident lesions in the field of ear, nose and throat.

3. Neck: Supple, no JVE, no LAP.

4. Chest: Bilateral clear breath sound, no wheezing or crackle were noted.

5. Heart: Regular heart beat, no murmurs.

6. Abdomen: Flat, normoactive bowel sound, tenderness over RUQ.
   Liver: 2 cm below the costal margin by percussion, impalpable.
   Spleen: Impalpable.
   Murphy's sign (+).

7. Extremities: Freely movable, no edema, ecchymosis, petechiae or rashes.

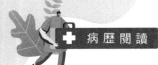

Laboratory:

1. CBC

Date	RBC	WBC	Hb	PLT	MCV	Hct	MCHC	MCH
2023/1/12	$4.50 \times 10^6/\mu L$	17,800/μL	13.0 g/dL	371,000/μL	94.0 fL	39.9%	34.1%	27.8 pg

2. Differential Count

Date	Neutrophils	Lymphocytes	Band form	Eosinophils	Monocytes	Basophils
2023/1/12	80.0%	22.0%	14.0%	1.0%	2.0%	0.0%

3. Coagulation

Date	PT	INR
2023/1/12	10 sec	1.0

4. BCS

Date	Glucose PC	BUN	Creatinine	Albumin	AST	ALT	LDH	TG	Sodium	Potassium
2023/1/12	110 mg/dL	17 mg/dL	0.7 mg/dL	3.0 g/dL	89 U/L	103 U/L	239 U/L	137 mg/L	139 mEq/L	3.9 mEq/L

Image Reports:

1. Abdominal ultrasound showed:
   (1) Dilatation of common bile duct proximal to the junction of common bile duct and main pancreatic duct.
   (2) Gallbladder thickening.
   (3) Bile slough in the gallbladder.
2. CT scan revealed:
   (1) A common bile duct stone obstruct the lumen of CBD.
   (2) Inflammatory change and thickening of the gallbladder.

Diagnosis:

Acute cholecystitis and a CBD stone.

Plan:

1. Antibiotic treatment, closely monitor the WBC count and the symptoms of abdominal pain to correlate with the response.

2. Give adequate hydration, IV fluid 2,200 mL/day run on a rate of 92 mL/hr.

3. Consult general surgeon and discuss the timing of receiving an operation.

Attending Physician: ×××

Resident: △△△

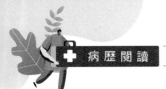

Progress Note

Hepatology and Gastroenterology, 54 years old, female, married, dormitory administrator.

Date of admission: 2023-1-12.

2023-1-12 10:00 am

#1 Acute cholecystitis, CBD stone

S: Mild fever, RUQ pain.

O: RUQ tenderness, Murphy's sign(+), WBC: 17,800/μL, AST: 89 U/L, ALT: 103 U/L.

A: Acute cholecystitis, CBD stone.

P:

1. Keep NPO & antibiotic treatment.

2. F/U bilirubin, ALP level.

3. Consult GS (general surgery) for op evaluation.

2 HTN

S: No headache, no chest pain.

O: BP: 160/95 mmHg.

A: Essential HTN.

P: Adalat 1# TID SL.

Attending Physician: ×××

Resident: △△△

Order Sheet

Hepatology and Gastroenterology, 54 years old, female, married, dormitory administrator.

Date of admission: 2023-1-12.

Standing Order

2023-1-12

Diagnosis:

1. Gallstones with acute cholecystitis.

2. CBD stone.

3. HTN.

Activity: Bed rest.

Allergies: Unknown.

Take BP, PR, RR QID.

NPO except medication.

Medications:

1. IVF with Taita No.5 1,200 mL + N/S 1,000 mL QD.

2. Cefmetazole 1g Q8H IV drip.

3. Scanol 1# QID PO.

4. Buscopan 1# QID PO.

5. Adalat 1# TID SL.

Attending Physician: ×××

Resident: △△△

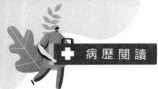

Stat Order

1. Check CBC+D/C, Bilirubin, ALP (CM).

2. Consult GS.

Attending Physician: ✕✕✕

Resident: △△△

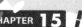
Ultrasound Requisition Sheet

日期	2023-1-12	病歷號碼	×××××
姓名	×××	醫師代碼	×××××

The applications:

☐ Spleen   ☐ Kidney   ■ Biliary Tree

☐ Abdominal Aorta   ☐ Thyroid   ☐ Liver

☐ Pancreas   ☐ Adrenal Gland   ☐ Prostate

☐ Carotid Echo   ☐ Other

Clinical data:

1. Murphy's sign (+).

2. WBC: 17,800/μL, AST: 89 U/L, ALT: 103 U/L.

Clinical diagnosis:

1. Acute cholecystitis.

2. CBD stone.

Report:

1. Dilatation of common bile duct proximal to the junction of common bile duct and main pancreatic duct.

2. Gallbladder thickening.

3. Bile slough in the gallbladder.

Physicion：×××

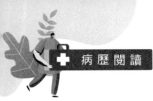
Consultation Sheet

姓名：○○○	病歷號碼：××××	床號：××	出生日期：****-*-*
性別：女	入院日期：2023-1-12	開單科別：肝膽胃腸科	照會科別：一般外科

The 54 year-old female, with HTN and hyperlipidemia has suffered from acute abdominal pain for one day. Abdominal echo revealed acute cholecystitis & CBD stone. Please kindly give your expert opinion on the surgical indication for the patient. Thanks a lot.

Dr. ××× at 2023-1-12 10:30 a.m.

Reply Sheet

Dear Dr.×××,

This is a case of gallstones & CBD stone with acute cholecystitis. Laparoscopic cholecystectomy & choledocholithotomy were suggested but patient hesitated. Please keep current treatment and consider endoscopic retrograde cholangiopancreatography for management of CBD stone. Many thanks for your consultation.

Dr.○○○ at 2023-1-12 2:30 p.m.

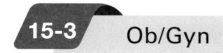

Ob/Gyn

Admission Note

Ob/Gyn, female, 54 years old, Taipei.

Information resource: The patient.

Chief Complaint:

Lower abdominal pain for about two months.

Present Illness:

This 54 year-old woman has suffered from lower abdominal pain since last November. The maximal pain intensity was located around her pubis. It exacerbated especially after urination, and persisted for about 5 minutes and often made her restlessness and very uncomfortable. No abnormal bleeding, vaginal spotting, nor dysmenorrhea were noticed. She visited local gynecologic clinic and ultrasonography showed 4 myomas in her uterus. She then went to another medical center and the result of the ultrasonography also revealed 4 uterine myomas. Via the recommendation of her friend, she came to our hospital and received ultrasonography again and revealed 4 uterine myomas, with the largest one measuring about 6 cm in diameter. Because of the bothering symptom of pain, surgical intervention was recommended and she was admitted to obstetric ward.

Ob/Gyn History:

1. Pregnancy history: G_3P_3, all NSD.
2. Menstruation history:
   (1) LMP: Around 12/21.
   (2) Last time previous to LMP was six months ago.

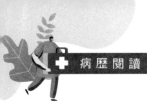

Past History:

1. Systemic diseases:
   (1) DM: 10+ years, the blood sugar is controlled by OHA and Insulin.
   (2) Hypertension: Duration is unspecified but is shorter than DM. BP is under medication control.
   (3) Hypercholestrolemia: Under medical control.
2. Operation history: Denied.
3. Current medication:
   (1) Glucophage 500 mg 2# BID PO.
   (2) Zocor 20 mg 1# HS QD PO.
   (3) Tanatril 5 mg 1# QD PO.
   (4) Hydrochlorothiazide 50 mg 0.5# QD PO.
   (5) Lantus solution 24 U HS QD SC.
   (6) Novorapid 3 U TID AC SC.

Family History:

1. Father died of complication of DM (unspecified complication).
2. Others are non-contributory.

Physical Examination:

1. Vital signs: BT: 36.5℃, PR: 85/min, RR: 14/min, BP: 130/84 mmHg.
2. General appearance: Well. Height: 156 cm, weight: 60 kg.
3. Consciousness: Clear; alert and oriented.
4. HEENT: Grossly normal; conjunctiva: Pinkish, not pale; sclera: anicteric.
5. Neck: Supple, no lymphadenopathy, no JVE, no goiter.
6. Chest: Symmetric expansion and no deformity. Clear breath sounds, no adventitious breath sounds are found.
7. Heart: Regular heart beat with normal S_1 and S_2, no murmur, no S_3 gallop.
8. Abdomen: Soft, bowel sound: Normoactive.

9. Limbs: No edema, peripheral pulses were all intact.

10. Neurological system: Prompt pupillary light reflex, the sensation of limbs are intact (no paresthesia).

Pelvic Examination:

1. Vulva: Grossly normal.

2. Vaginal discharge: Clear.

3. Vaginal: Grossly normal, no lesions are noted.

4. Cervix: Smooth, the discharge is also clear.

5. Uterus: AVFL, hypertrophy.

6. Adnexa: Free.

Laboratory:

1. CBC

Date	RBC	WBC	Hb	Platelet	MCV	HCT	MCHC	MCH
2023/3/10	4.00 M /uL	7,200/uL	13.0 g/dL	301,000/uL	96.5fL	44.1%	33.1 g/dL	29.1 pg

2. Differential Count

Date	Neutrophil	Lymphocyte	Band form	Eosinophil	Monocyte	Basophil
2023/3/10	78%	14%	2%	1%	5%	0.0%

3. Coagulation

Date	PT	INR
2023/3/10	12 sec	0.9

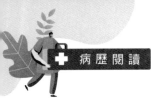

4. BCS

Date	Glucose (PC)	BUN	Creatinine	AST	Albumin	ALT	Sodium
2023/3/10	160 mg/dL	22 mg/dL	1.0 mg/L	30 U/L	3.0 g/dL	23 U/L	141 mEq/L
	TG	Potassium					
	170 mg/L	5.0 mEq/L					

Image Study:

Transvaginal ultrasound reveals 2 myomas located at the posterior uterine wall, 1 myoma is 4 cm in diameter and is near the angle, the other one is 6 cm in diameter at the Douglas pouch.

Tentative Diagnosis:

Multiple uterine myomas.

Therapeutic Plans:

1. Prepare for subtotal hysterectomy.
2. Blood sugar and pressure control.
3. Anesthesiologist consultation.

Attending Physician: ×××

Resident: △△△

15-4 **Gastroenterology**

Admission Note

Gastroenterology, male , 24 years old, Taichung.

Date of admission: 2023-1-12.

Chief Complaint:

Severe abdominal pain for 3 days.

Present Illness:

This 24 year-old patient was quite healthy before until he had abdominal pain 3 days previous to this admission. The pain first presented after meals with a dull, continuous feature. It was located at the central abdomen, and would exacerbated when he was in a supine position and relieved when bending forward. He took antacids but it did not relieved. However, the intensity of pain reduced when he didn't eat anything. On the day of admission, he felt too painful to get to the school; thus, he went to our ER.

At the ER, he looked very sick but the vital signs were still stable. He didn't vomit, feel nauseous, pass blood stool or have diarrhea. His mucosal surface was dry. Physical examination revealed severe, diffuse tenderness over the abdomen with the most intense point located around the umbilicus. There was no rebound tenderness. The Mcbourney sign and Murphy's sign were both negative. Cardiac and chest examinations showed no abnormalities.

Under the impression of acute pancreatitis, he was admitted and asked for NPO.

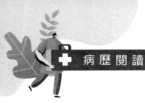

Past History:

1. Systemic disease: AIDS(-), HBV(-), HCV(-), COPD(-), gout(-), CVA(-), DM(-), HTN(-), hyperlipidemia(-), gallstone(-).
2. Hospitalization: Denied.
3. Operation: Denied.
4. Medication: Denied.
5. Alcohol consumption: Denied.
6. Smoking: Denied.
7. Betel nut: Denied.
8. Allergic history: Denied.

Family History:

1. Mother: Breast cancer s/p right mastectomy + adjuvant chemotherapy (5 years ago).
2. Father: BPH s/p TUR-BP 2 years ago.
3. Elder brother: Asthma since he was born.

Physical Examination:

1. General appearance: Acute-illness, consciousness: Clear. BW: 68 kg, BH: 176 cm.
2. Vital sign: BP: 140/92 mmHg, BT: 37.7℃, PR: 90/min, RR: 18/min.
3. HEENT: Pinkish conjunctiva, anicteric sclera, no gum bleeding, no tonsillar enlargement, no throat injection, pupillary light reflex: Prompt and symmetric in both eyes. The mucosal surface of eyes and oral cavity were dry.
4. Neck: Supple. No jugular vein engorgement, no palpable lymph node, normal sized thyroid gland. No carotid bruit.
5. Chest and lungs: Symmetric expansion. Clear breath sound. No crackles, wheeze or stridor. His breaths were relative rapid and shallow.
6. Heart: Regular heart beats, no murmur, normal S_1 and S_2, no S_3 or S_4.

7. Abdomen: Flat, hypoactive bowel sound, no shifting dullness, severe tenderness all over the abdomen with the most painful point around his umbilicus, no rebound tenderness, normal liver and spleen size by percussion and palpation. Mcbourney sign(-), Murphy's sign(-).

8. Extremities: No deformity, free joint movement. No edema.

9. Peripheral pulsations: Normal and equal in carotid, brachial, popliteal and dorsalis pedis arteries.

10. Neurologic examination: Clear and alert consciousness, oriented and coherent to time, place and person. No abnormal cranial nerve signs. No sensory function deficit. No motor deficit. No urinary or fecal incontinence, no constipation or diarrhea.

Laboratory:

1. CBC

Date	RBC	WBC	Hb	Platelet	MCV	HCT	MCHC	MCH
2023/1/12	5.50 M/uL	21,000/uL	15.1 g/dL	280,000/uL	93.1 fL	45%	35.0 g/dL	26.6 pg

2. Differential count

Date	Neutrophil	Lymphocyte	Monocyte	Eosinophil	Basophil
2023/1/12	90%	8%	1%	0.5%	0.5%

3. BCS

Date	Glucose (PC)	BUN	Creatinine	AST	Amylase
2023/1/12	120 mg/dL	30 mg/dL	1.1 mg/L	60 U/L	500 U/L
	Serum lipase	K	T-bilirubin	Na	—
	300 U/L	3.6 mEq/L	2.5 mg/dL	145 mEq/L	—

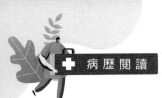
Diagnosis:

Acute pancreatitis.

Therapeutic Plans:

1. NPO.
2. Narcotic analgesics.
3. Adequate hydration.

Attending Physician: ✕ ✕ ✕

Resident: △△△

Metabolism

Admission Note

Metabolism, female, 25 years old, Yilan.

Source of information: The patient.

Date of admission: 2023-2-12.

Chief Complaint:

Intermittent palpitation for 2 months.

Present Illness:

This 25 year-old female was presented to our emergency department (ED) complaining of intermittent palpitations for 2 months. The palpitations were episodic even at rest. There was no obvious precipitating factor. In addition, she had reported insomnia, heat-intolerance, tremor, increased frequency of defecation, and a 6 kg weight loss despite having a good appetite. There was no fever, chills, changed consciousness, chest pain, vomiting, tarry stool, or proximal muscular weakness. The patient denied taking diuretics[5] or other medicine.

On arrival at the ED, she looked anxious with shortness of breath. Initial investigation showed her pulse around 110 beats/minute, blood pressure around 148/90 mmHg, respiratory rate around 24/minute, and body temperature around 36℃. The 12-lead ECG revealed sinus tachycardia, and the CXR showed no remarkable findings. Due to goiter and proptosis, her blood was sampled to check thyroid function. After initial evaluation and management, she was suggested to be admitted for further work up and treatment.

Past History:

1. Systemic diseases: Denied.
2. Hospitalization: Denied.

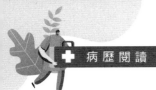

3. Operaton: Denied.

4. Medication: Denied.

5. Alcohol consumption: Denied.

6. Smoking: Denied.

7. Betel nut: Denied.

8. Allergic history: Denied.

Family History:

1. Mother had goiter s/p partial thyroidectomy 10 years ago.

2. Elder sister has hypothyroidism under Elthoxin supplement for the past one year.

Physical Examination:

1. General appearance: Anxious. BH: 160 cm, BW: 45 kg. BP: 140/86 mmHg, PR: 100/min, RR: 20/min, BT: 36.4℃.

2. HEENT: Proptosis (OU), no anemic conjunctiva, anicteric sclera, no throat injection. No grossly evident lesions in the field of ear and nose.

3. Neck: Goiter with thrill and bruit, supple, no jugular vein engorgement, no palpable LN.

4. Chest and lungs: Symmetric expansion. Resonance on percussion in all lung fields. Bil. clear breathing sounds. No wheeze, no crackle.

5. Heart: Rapid heart beats.

6. Abdomen: Soft and flat, hyperactive bowel sound, no tenderness, no shifting dullness, normal liver and spleen size by percussion and palpation.

7. Extremitis: Warm and moist, free joint movement, mild non-pitting edema over bil. lower legs, no deformity.

8. Neurologic examination: Clear and alert consciousness, no abnormal cranial nerve signs, no abnormal sensory function, no motor deficit.

Laboratory:

Date	WBC	Neutrophil	Lymphocyte	Eosinophil	Hb	MCV	Platelet
2023-2-12	5,600/μL	70%	18%	3%	12.8 g/dL	88.4 fL	240000/μL
	Glucose	**ALT**	**Creatinine**	**Na**	**K**	**TSH**	**Free T$_4$**
	98/mg/dL	36 IU/L	1.0 mg/dL	136 mEq/L	3.2 mEqL	0.00 μIU/mL	4.00 ng/dL

Impression:

Goiter.

Therapeutic Plans:

1. Arrange subtotal thyroidectomy.
2. Post-OP Levothyroxine (50 mcg) 1 #　QD　PO.

Attending Physician: ×××

Resident: △△△

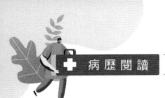
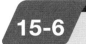
15-6 Orthopedic

Admission Note

Orthopedic department, 65 years old, female, married, housewife.

Date of admission: 2023-4-12.

Chief Complaint:

Left knee pain for several years.

Present Illness:

This 65 year-old woman without underlying disease has suffered from pain while walking in both knees. The pain was worse in her left knee than in her right knee. She had received conservative treatment in the past. Recently, she felt the pain in both knees was getting worse day by day. It was difficult to walk and unable to climb stairs or squat. One time at our OPD, X-ray of both knees revealed joint space narrowing with genu varus deformity and osteophyte formation. Physical examination disclosed joint effusion, instability, varus deformity. As surgical intervention was suggested, she was admitted for left total knee replacement (TKR) surgery.

Past History:

1. Occupation: Housewife.

2. No DM or hypertension history in the past.

3. Smoking history: No smoking habit.

4. Alcohol history: No alcohol consumption habit.

5. The history of major operation: Nil.

6. No known food or drug allergy.

Personal History:

1. Habit of smoking: Denied.

2. Habit of alcohol drinking: Denied.

3. The history of occupation disease: Nil.

4. The history of traveling in recent 3 months: Denied.

5. The history of drug abuse: Denied.

Family History:

Nothing in particular.

Review of Systems:

Throughout the whole course of present illness, the patient also suffered from symptoms mentioned as below: Chills(-), fever(-), night sweating(-), cough(-), sputum(-), hemoptysis(-), epistaxis(-), chest tightness(-), chest pain(-), SOB(-), exertional dyspnea(-), orthopnea(-), abdominal pain(-), anorexia(-), dysphagia(-), nausea(-), vomiting(-), constipation(-), diarrhea(-), hematemesis(-), hematochezia(-), melena(-), dysuria(-), oligouria(-), body weight loss(-).

1. Vital signs: BT: 36.6°C, PR: 72/min, RR: 24~26/min, BP: 142/86mmHg.

2. Height: 163 cm, Weight: 66 kg.

3. Conscious: Alert.

4. Mentality: Intact to JOMAC.

5. Skin: No petechiae or ecchymosis, dry skin turgor.

6. HEENT: Grossly normal, no pale conjunctiva or icteric sclera.

7. Neck: Supple, no jugular vein engorgement, no goiter.

8. Chest: Symmetrical and free expansion, breathing sound(-).

9. Heart: Regular heart beat, no murmur, no heave or no thrill.

10. Abdomen: Soft and flat, normoactive bowel sound, no shifting dullness, no tenderness or rebounding pain.

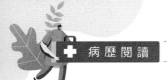

11. Back: No spine deformity, no CV angle knocking pain.

12. Extremities: Freely movable, bilateral genu varus deformity, left knee contracture with mild limitation of extension.

13. Neurological: Limbs sensory, motion: Intact.

Laboratory:

1. BCS

Date	Glucose PC	BUN	Creatinine	AST	ALK-P	Albumin	Sodium	Potassium
2023/4/1	123 dL	36 mg/dL	1.0 dL	10 U/L	70 U/L	4.5 L	134 mEq/L	4 q/L

2. CBC

Date	WBC	RBC	Hb	Hct	MCV	PLT	Neutrophils	Monocytes	Basophils
2023/4/1	7,400 μL	4.39×10^6/μL	14 g/dL	41%	87 fL	292,000 μL	70.2%	7.5%	2.4%

3. 2023-3-25 Biltaeral knee X ray

Imaging findings:

Both knees and Marchant view shows: Joint space narrowing with spurs formation, compatible with osteoarthritis, bilateral mild genu deformity, and left marginal spur of left patella.

Impression:

Left knee OA.

Plans:

1. Left total knee replacement.
2. Post-op care and rehabilitation.

Attending Physician: ×××

Resident: △△△

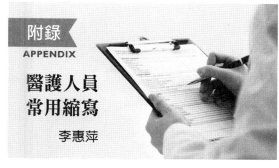

附錄
APPENDIX

醫護人員
常用縮寫
李惠萍

A

aa or a	每一，各一	
AAA	Abdominal aorta aneurysm　腹主動脈瘤	
AAD	Against-advice discharge　自動出院	
Ab	Abortion　墮胎	
ABE	Acute bacterial endocarditis 急性細菌性心內膜炎	
ABG	Arterial blood gas　動脈血液氣體	
AC	(L. *ante cibum*, before meal)　飯前	
ACE	Angiotensin-converting enzyme 血管收縮素轉換酶	
ACJ	Dislocation　acromiolaviculat joint dislocation　肩鎖關節脫臼	
ACL	Anterior cruciate ligament 前十字韌帶	
ACOA	Adult children of alcoholics 成人兒童酒癮患者	
ACVD	Acutecardiovascular disease 急性心血管疾病	
AD	(L. *Auris Dextra*, right ear)　右耳	
ad., add	(L. *adde,* addition)　加，加到	
ad.lib.	(L. *Ad libitum*, at will)　隨意	
ADH	Antidiuretic hormone　抗利尿激素	
ADHD	Attention deficit hyperactivity disorder 注意力不足／過動症	
ADL	Activeites of daily living　日常生活活動	
ADM	Admission　入院，住院	

AE	Above the elbow　肘上方	
Af	Atrial fibrillation　心房纖維性顫動	
AF	Atrial flutter　心房撲動	
AFB	*Acid-fast bacillus*　嗜酸桿菌	
AFE	Amniotic fluid embolism　羊水栓塞	
A/G	Albumin/globulin ratio　白蛋白／球蛋白比率	
AG	Abdominal girth　腹圍	
AGE	Acute gastroenteritis　急性腸胃炎	
AGML	Acute gastric mucosal lesion 急性胃黏膜受損	
AGN	Acute glomerulonephritis　急性腎絲球腎炎	
AHN	Assistant head nurse　副護理長	
AI	Aortic insufficiency　主動脈瓣閉鎖不全	
AIDS	Acquired immunodeficiency syndrome　後天性免疫不全症候群（愛滋病）	
AJ	Ankle jerk　踝反射	
AK	Above the knee　膝上方	
ALD	Adrenoleukodystrophy　腎上腺腦白質退化症	
ALL	Acute lymphocytic leukemia 急性淋巴性白血病	
ALS	Amyotrophic lateral sclerosis 肌萎縮性脊髓側索硬化症	
ALT	Alanine aminotransferase　麩胺基酸焦葡萄轉胺基酶	
AM	(L. *Ante meridiem*, before noon) 上午	
AMI	Acute myocardial infarction 急性心肌梗塞	
amp	Ampule　安瓿	
AN	Associate nurse　助理護士	
ANS	Autonomic nervous system　自主神經系統	
AOD	Arterial occlusive disease 動脈阻塞疾病	
AP	Antepartum　分娩前的；懷孕	
~	Anterior to posterior　由前至後	

APC	Atrial premature contraction 心房性早期收縮	
APH	Antepartum hemorrhage　產前出血	
APR	Abdominal perineal resection 腹部會陰切除術	
Aq	(L. *Aqua*, water)　水	
AR	Aortic regurgitation　主動脈逆流	
ARF	Acute renal failure　急性腎衰竭	
~	Acute respiratory failure　急性呼吸衰竭	
AROM	Artificial ROM　人工破水	
AS	Aortic stenosis　主動脈狹窄	
~	Arteriosclerosis　動脈粥樣硬化	
~	(L. *Auris ainistra*, left ear)　左耳	
ASCVD	Arteriosclerotic cardiovascular disease　動脈硬化的心血管疾病	
ASD	Atrial septal defect　心房中隔缺損	
ASHD	Arteriosclerotic heart disease 動脈硬化性心臟病	
AST	Abdominal tubal sterilization 腹式輸卵管絕育術	
AT	Aerosol therapy　噴霧吸入療法	
ATH	Abdominal total hysterectomy　腹式全子宮切除術	
ATP	Adenosine triphosphate　腺苷三磷酸	
AU	(L. *Auris uterque*, both ears)　雙耳	
AV block	Artrioventricular block　心房心室傳導阻斷	
AV shunt	Arteriovenous shunt 動靜脈分流	
AVM	Arteriovenous malformation 動靜脈畸形	
AVN	Avascular necrosis　缺血性壞死	
AVNFH	Avascular necrosis of femoral head 股骨頭缺血性壞死	

B

BAEP	Brain-stem autitory evoked potential 腦幹聽力誘發電位
BAVP	Balloon aortic valvuloplasty 主動脈瓣氣球擴張術

BB	Blood bank　血庫
BBBB	Bilateral bundle branch block 雙側束支傳導阻滯
BBT	Basal body temperature　基礎體溫
B&C	Biopsy and curettage　組織切片與刮除術
B/C	Blood culture　血液培養
B/C, BUN/Cr.	Blood urea nitrogen/creatinine ratio 血尿素氮及肌酸酐比率
BCA	Balloon catheter angioplasty 氣球導管血管整形術
BCC	Basal cell carcinoma　基底細胞癌
BCG	Bacille Calmette-Guérin　卡介苗
BCU	Burn care unit　燒傷中心
BD	Birth date　出生日期
~	Brain death　腦死
BE	Barium enema　鋇劑灌腸
~	Below the elbow　肘下方
BH	Body height　身高
BICU	Baby intensive care unit　嬰兒加護中心
BID	(L. *Bis in die*, twice a day)　每天兩次
Bil	Bilateral　雙側的
BIN	(L. *Bis in nocte*, twice a night) 每夜兩次
BIOP, Bx	Biopsy　活體組織切片
BK	Below the knee　膝下方
BLS	Basic life support　基本救命術
BM	Bowel movement　腸蠕動
BMA	Bone marrow aspiration　骨髓抽吸
BMR	Basal metabolic rate　基礎代謝率
BP	Blood pressure　血壓
BPB	Blood platelet count　血小板計數
BPD	Biparietal diameter　雙頂間徑

BPH	Benign prostatic hypertrophy 良性前列腺肥大		**CCF**	Congestive cardiac failure　充血性心衰竭
BPLA	Bilateral pelvic lympho adenectomy 兩側骨盆淋巴腺切除術		**Ccr.**	Creatinine clearance rate　肌酸酐廓清率
BR	Baby room　嬰兒室		**CCU**	Cardiology care unit　心臟病加護中心
Brain CT	Brain computerized tomography 腦部電腦斷層攝影		~	Coronary care unit　冠狀動脈疾病加護中心
BSA	Body surface area　身體表面積		**CDCR**	Conjunctiva dacryocystorhinotomy 結合膜淚囊鼻腔切開術
BSO	Bilateral salpingo-oophorectomy 雙側輸卵管卵巢切除術		**CDH**	Congenital dislocation of the hip 先天性髖關節脫臼
BT	Bleeding time　出血時間		**CE**	Cardiac enlargement　心臟擴大
~	Blood transfusion　輸血		~	Cerebral edema　腦水腫
BTI	Biliary tract infection　膽道感染		**CFS**	Chronic fatigue syndrome　慢性疲勞症候群
BUS	Blood, urine, stool(routine) 血液、尿液及糞便（常規檢查）		**CGN**	Chronic glomerulonephritis　慢性腎絲球腎炎
BW	Body weight　體重		**CH**	Cerebral hemorrhage　腦出血
Bx	Biopsy　活組織檢查		**chart.** or **cht.**	(L. *Chartula*, paper)　病歷

C

C	Celsius, centigrade, complement　攝氏，百分度，補體		**CHD**	Congenital heart disease　先天性心臟病
Ca	Calcium cancer, Carcinoma 鈣，癌症		**CHD**	Congenital hip dislocation　先天性髖脫位
CABG	Coronary artery bypass graft 冠狀動脈繞道手術		~	Coronary heart disease　冠狀動脈性心臟病
CAD	Coronary artery disease　冠狀動脈疾病		**CHF**	Congestive heart failure　充血性心臟衰竭
cAMP	Cyclic adenosine monophosphate 環腺苷單磷酸		**CHR**	Chronic hypertrophy rhinitis 慢性肥厚性鼻炎
Cap.	Capsule　膠囊		**Ci.**	Curie　居里（放射性強度）
CAPD	Continuous ambulatory peritoneal dialysis　持續活動性腹膜透析		**CIN**	Cervical intra-epithelium neoplasm 內宮頸上皮腫瘤
cath	Catheter　導管		**CIS**	Carcinoma *in situ*　原位癌
CBC	Complete blood count　全血球計數		**CK**	Creatine kinase　肌酸激酶
CBD	Common bile duct　總膽管		**Cl**	Chloride, chlorine　氯
CC, C/O	Chief complaint　主訴		**cm**	Centimeter　公分
c.c.	Cubic centimeter　立方公分，毫升		**CM**	Coming morning　隔天早上
			CN	Charge nurse　負責護士
			~	Cras nocte, tomorrow night　明晚

CNM	Certified nurse midwife　合格護理助產士		~	Computed tomography(scan)　電腦斷層攝影
CNS	Central nervous system　中樞神經系統		**CTS**	Carpal tunnel syndrome　腕隧道症候群
CO	Cardiac output　心輸出量		**CU**	Convalescent unit　恢復室
CO₂	Carbon dioxide　二氧化碳		**CUR**	Curettage　擴創
Collut.	(L. *Collutorium*, mouth wash)　漱口劑		**CVA**	Cerebrovascular accident, stroke　腦血管意外，中風
Collyr.	(L. *Collyrium*, eyewash)　洗眼劑		**CVD**	Cardiovascular disease　心血管疾病

CO₂ — Carbon dioxide　二氧化碳

COM	Chronic otitis media　慢性中耳炎
COPD	Chronic obstructive pulmonary disease　慢性阻塞性肺病
CP	Cerebral palsy　腦性麻痺
CPA	Cardiopulmonary arrest　心肺停止
CPD	Cephalopelvic disproportion　胎頭與骨盆不相稱
CPK	Creatine phosphokinase(cardiac enzyme)　肌酸磷酸激酶
CPK-MB	Creatine phosphokinase muscle band isoenzyme　肌酸磷酸激酶－橫紋肌型同功異構酶
CPR	Cardiopulmonary resuscitation　心肺復甦術
CPS	Chronic paranasal sinusitis　慢性鼻竇炎
CPT	Chest physiotherapy　胸腔物理治療
CR	Chief resident　總住院醫師
CRF	Chronic renal failure　慢性腎衰竭
CS	Consultation　會診
C/S	Cesarean section　剖腹生產
C&S	Culture and sensitivity (antibiotic susceptibility)　培養與敏感試驗
CSF	Cerebrospinal fluid　腦脊髓液
CSR	Central supply room　中央供應中心
~	Cervical spinal radiculopathy　頸脊髓神經根病
CSW	Certified social worker　合格社會工作者
CT	Cerebral thrombosis　腦血栓
~	Chemotherapy　化學療法，化療

CVP	Central venous pressure　中心靜脈壓
CVS	Cardiovascular surgery　心臟血管外科
~	Chorionic villi sampling　絨毛取樣
CXR	Chest X-ray　胸部 X 光攝影

D

DAS	Died at scene　當場死亡
DB	Deep breathe　深呼吸
DB, DOB	Date of birth　出生日期
D&C	Dilation and curettement　擴張及刮除術（人工流產）
DC	Discharge　出院
~	Discontinue　停止
DCC	Day care center　日間照護中心
DCM	Dilated cardiomyopathy　擴張型心肌病變
DCR	Dacryocystorhinostomy　淚囊鼻腔造瘻術
DD	Discharge diagnosis　出院診斷
DDH	Developed dysplasia of hip　髖關節發育不良
DDS	Doctor of dental surgery(dentist)　牙醫
DDx	Differential diagnosis　鑑別診斷
D&E	Dilatation and evacuation　擴張與抽吸術
Dent.	Dentology　牙科
Derm	Dermatology　皮膚科
dexter	Dexter　右
DHS	Duration of hospital stay　住院期間
DIC	Diffuse intravascular coagulation　瀰漫性血管內凝血

dil. Dilue, dilutus　稀釋

DIP Distal inter phalangeal　遠端指骨間

DJD Degenerative joint disease　變性關節疾病

DKA Diabetic ketoacidosis　糖尿病酮症酸中毒

dl Deciliter　十分之一公升

DM Diabetes mellitus　糖尿病

DMS Diagnostic medical sonography　醫學超音波診斷

DNA Deoxyribonucleic acid　去氧核醣核酸

DND Died a natural death　自然死亡

DNR Do not resuscitate　不予施行心肺復甦術

DNS Deviation of nasal septum　鼻中隔彎曲

DOD Date of death　死亡日期

DON Director of nursing　護理部主任

DOS Date of surgery　手術日期

dos. (L. *Dosis*, dosage)　劑量

DR Delivery room　產房

DRG Diagnostic-related group　診斷相關組

D/T Diet therapy　飲食療法

DTaP-Hib-IPV Diphtheria and tetanus toxoid with acellular pertussis, inactivated polio and *haemophilus influenzae* type b vaccine　五合一疫苗（白喉、破傷風、非細胞性百日咳、b型嗜血桿菌及不活化小兒麻痺混合疫苗）

DTR Deep tendon reflex　深部肌腱反射

DTs Delirium tremens　震顫性譫妄

DU Duodenal ulcer　十二指腸潰瘍

DUB Dysfunctional uterine bleeding　功能失常性子宮出血

DVT Deep vein thrombosis　深部靜脈栓塞

D/W Dextrose in water　葡萄糖水

Dx Diagnosis　診斷

E

EA Epidural anesthesia　硬膜外麻醉法

ECCE Extracapsular cataract extraction　白內障囊外摘除術

ECF Extracellular fluid　細胞外液

ECG, EKG Electrocardiogram　心電圖

ECHO Echocardiogram　心臟超音波

~ Echoencephalogram　腦部超音波

ECLE Extracapsular lens extraction　水晶體囊外摘除術

ECN Extended care nursery　加護育嬰室

ECT Eelectroconvulsive therapy　電休克治療

EDC Expected date of confinement　預產期

EEG Electroencephalogram　腦電圖，腦波圖

EFW Estimated fetal weight　估計胎兒體重

EGD Esophagogastroduodenoscopy　食道胃十二指腸鏡檢

EMG Electromyogram　肌電圖

EMT Emergency medical technician　救護技術員

ENDO Endoscopy　內視鏡檢查

ENT Ear nose and throat　耳鼻喉

EOD Every other day　每隔一天

EOM Extraocular movement　眼球外轉運動

EP Episiotomy　女陰切開術

~ Evoked potential　誘發電位

EPS Extra pyramidal sndrome　椎體外症候群

ER Emergency room　急診室

ERCP Endoscopic retrograde cholangiopancreatography　逆行性胰膽管內視鏡造影術

ESD Emergency services department　急診部

ESR Erythrocyte sedimentation rate　紅血球沉降速率

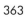

ESRD	End-Stage Renal Disease　末期腎病	
ESWL	Extracorporeal shock wave lithotripsy 體外震波碎石術	
ET	Electrotherapy　電治療	
ETGA	Endotracheal general anesthesia 氣管內全身麻醉	
EVL	Esophageal varices ligation　食道靜脈曲張結紮	

F

°F	Fahrenheit degrees　華氏（溫度）
F	Female　雌的，女（性）的
FAS	Fetal alcohol syndrome　胎兒酒精症候群
FBS	Fasting blood sugar　空腹血糖
FDA	Food and Drug Administration　食品藥物管理局
FH	Family history　家族史
FHB	Fetal heart beat　胎兒心跳
FHS	Fetal heart sound　胎兒心音
FiO₂	Fraction of inspired oxygen　吸入氧氣份量
FM	Fetal movement　胎動
FSD	Fundal symphysis distance　胃底恥骨距離
FSH	Follicle-stimulating hormone 濾泡刺激素
Ft	Foot, feet (measure)　英尺（測量單位）
FUO	Fever of unknown origin　不明原因發燒
Fr.	Fracture　骨折
Fx.	Frozen section　冷凍切片

G

G	Gravida　孕次
G, g	Gram　公克
G-6-PD	Glucose-6-phosphate dehydrogenase 葡萄糖-6-磷酸去氫酶
GA	General anesthesia　全身麻醉

garg.	Gargarisma　漱口
GBD	Gallbladder stone　膽囊結石
GCS	Glasgow coma scale　格拉斯哥氏昏迷指數
GDM	Gestational diabetes mellitus 妊娠期糖尿病
gel.	Gelatum　凝膠
GERD	Gastroesophageal reflux disease 胃食道逆流症
GFR	Glomerular filtration rate 腎絲球過濾速率
GHB	Glycated hemoglobin　糖化血色素
GI	Gastrointestinal　胃腸
GIFT	Gamete intrafallopian tube transfer 禮物嬰兒，試管嬰兒
GITT	Glucose-insulin tolerance test 葡萄糖胰島素耐受性試驗
GLU	Glucose　葡萄糖
GMR	General medical routine　一般內科常規
GSR	General surgical routine　一般外科常規
GTT	Glucose tolerance test　葡萄糖耐量試驗
gtt.	(L. *Gutta*, a drop of water)　滴
GU	Genitourinary　泌尿生殖器
Gy	Gray　蒼白
Gyn	Gynecology　婦科

H

H	Hormone　荷爾蒙
HA	Headache　頭痛
HAV	Hepatits A virus　A 型肝炎病毒
Hb.	Hemoglobin　血紅素
HbA₁c	Hemoglobin A₁c(test)　糖化血色素
HBV	Hepatitis B virus　B 型肝炎病毒
HCC	Hepatocellular carcinoma　肝細胞性肝癌
hCG	Human chorionic gonadotropin 人類絨毛膜性腺激素

HCl	Hydrochloric acid, hydrochloride 鹽酸;氯化氫
HCO₃⁻	Bicarbonate 重碳酸鹽
Hct	Hematocrit 血比容
HCVD	Hypertensive cardiovascular Disease 高血壓性心臟病
HD	Heart disease 心臟病
~	Hemodialysis 血液透析
HDL	High-density lipoprpteins 高密度脂蛋白
HDU	Hemodialysis unit 血液透析室
Hg	Mercury 汞,水銀
HHD	Hypertensive heart disease 高血壓性心臟病
HIV	Human immunodeficiency virus 人類免疫缺失病毒
HIVD	Herniated intervertebral disc 椎間盤脫出
HLA	Human leukocyte antigen 人類白血球抗原
HN	Head nurse 護理長
HP	*Helicobacter pylori.* 幽門螺旋桿菌
HPV	Human papillomavirus 人類乳頭狀瘤病毒
HR	Heart rate 心跳速率
hr.	Hour 小時
h.s.	(L.*Hora somni*, at bed time) 睡前
HSG	Hysterosalpingogram 子宮輸卵管攝影
HSV	Herpes simplex virus 單純疱疹病毒
H/T	Hypertension 高血壓
Ht	Hypodermic tablet 皮下錠
Hx	History 歷史,經歷
Hypo.	Hypodermic (injection) 皮下的(注射)
Hz	Hertz 赫茲(頻率單位:周/秒)

I

I&D	Incision and Drainage 切開及引流
I&O	Intake and Output 攝入和輸出

i.c.	Inter cibus 兩餐間
IABP	Intra-aortic balloon pump 動脈內氣球幫浦
IBS	Irritable bowel syndrome 腸躁症
IC	Intracutaneous(injection)皮內的(注射)
ICF	Intracellular fluid 細胞內液
ICH	Intracerebral hemorrhage 顱內出血
ICN	Infection control nurse 感染控制護理人員
ICT	Intracerebral tumor 顱內腫瘤
ICU	Intensive care unit 加護病房
IDA	Iron deficiency anemia 缺鐵性貧血
IDK	Internal derangement knee 膝關節內障礙
IgA	Immunoglobin A 免疫球蛋白A
IGTT, IVGTT	Intravenous glucose tolerence test 靜脈注射葡萄糖耐受性試驗
IHD stone	Intra hepatic duct stone 內肝管結石
IICP	Increased intracranial pressure 顱內壓增高
IL	Interleukin 介白素
ILOC	Immediate loss of consciousness 立即喪失意識
IM	Intramuscular injection 肌肉內注射
INFH	Ischemic necrosis of femoral head 股骨頭缺血性壞死
inh	Inhallation 蒸氣吸入
IOFB	Intraocular foreign body 眼內異物
IOP	Intraocular pressure 眼內壓力
IPF	Idiopathic pulmonary fibrosis 特發性肺纖維化
IPPB	Intermittint positive pressure breathing 間歇性正壓呼吸
IT	Inhalation therapy 吸入療法
ITP	Idiopathic thrombocytopenic purpura 特發性血小板減少性紫斑
ITT	Insulin tolerance test 胰島素耐受性試驗

IU	International unit　國際單位	**lb**	Pound　英磅
IUD	Intrauterine device　子宮內避孕器	**LC**	Laparoscopic cholecystectomy　腹腔鏡膽囊切除術
IUFD	Intrauterine fetal death　胎兒宮內死亡	~	Liver cirrhosis　肝硬化
IUGR	Intrauterine growth retardation　胎兒宮內發育遲緩	**LCL**	Lateral collateral ligament　外側副韌帶
IV drip	Intravenous drip　靜脈滴注	**LD**	Local dentist　地方開業牙醫
IVF	In vitro fertilization　體外受精	**LDH**	Lactic dehydrogenase　乳酸去氫酶
~	Intravenous fluid　靜脈輸液	**LFT**	Liver function test　肝功能試驗
IVI	Intravitreous injection　玻璃體內注射	**LGA**	Large for gestational age　胎兒體重過重
IVP	Intravenous pyelography　靜脈注射腎盂攝影	**lin.**	Linimentum　擦劑
IVU	Intravenous urography　靜脈尿道造影	**liq.**	Liquid　液體
		LLQ	(L. *Left lower quadrant*, abdomen)　左下腹部

J

JBE	Japanese B encephalitis　日本B型腦炎	**LMD**	Local medical doctor　地方開業醫師
JC	Junior clinicians　資淺臨床醫師	**LMP**	Last menstrual period　最後一次月經
		LOA	Left occiput anterior　左枕前位

K

		LOP	Left occiput posterior　左枕後位
K	Potassium　鉀	**LOT**	Left occiput transverse　左枕橫位
Kcal	Kilocalorie (food calorie)千卡（食物熱量）	**LOT**	Licensed occupational therapist　有執照之職能治療師
Kg	Kilogram　公斤	**lot.**	Lotion　乳液（擦劑）
km	Kilometer　公里	**LP**	Lumbar puncture　腰椎穿刺
KUB	Kidney, ureter, and bladder　腎、輸尿管及膀胱（腹部X光攝影）	**LPN**	Licensed practical nurse　有執照之領照執業護士
		LPO	Left posterior oblique　左後斜

L

L	Left　左邊	**LR**	Labor room　產房
~	Liter　公升	**LTT**	Lactose tolerance test　乳糖耐受性試驗
LA	Local anesthesia　局部麻醉	**LUQ**	Left upper quadrant(abdomen)　左上（腹）
Lapa	Laparotomy　剖腹手術	**LVN**	Licensed vocational nurse　有執照之職業護士
Laser	Light amplification by stimulated emission of radiation　光放大的激輻射		

M

LAVH	Laparoscopy abdominal vaginal hysterectomy　腹腔鏡陰式子宮切除術	**M**	Meter　公尺
		~	Molar　莫耳（分子單位）
		~	Male　男性的
		M&N	Morning and night　早晚

MAR	Medication administration record 給藥記錄		**mmHg**	Millimeters of mercury　毫米汞柱
MAS	Meconium aspiration syndrome 胎糞吸入症候群		**MMR**	Measles, Mumps, Rubella (vaccine) 麻疹，腮腺炎，風疹（疫苗）
mas.	(L. *Massa*, mass)　硬塊		**MN**	Midnight　半夜，午夜
MBD	May be discharged　核准出院		**MOD**	Notify of death　宣布死亡
~	Minimal brain dysfunction　輕度腦障礙		**MR**	Mitral regurgitation　二尖瓣逆流
			MRD	Medical record department　病歷室
mcg, μg	Microgram　微克（百萬分之一公克）		**MRI**	Magnetic resonance imaging 核磁共振造影
MCH	Mean corpuscular hemoglobin　平均血球血紅素		**MS**	Meconium stain　胎便染色
			~	Mitral stenosis　二尖瓣狹窄
MCHC	Mean corpuscular hemoglobin concentration　平均血球血紅素濃度		~	Multiple sclerosis　多發性硬化症
			MSA	Multiple system atrophy　多重系統退化
MCL	Medial collateral ligament　內側副韌帶		**MSE**	Mental status examination 心智狀態檢查
~	Middle cruciate ligament　內十字韌帶		**MT**	Medical technologist　醫療技師
MCV	Mean corpuscular volume　平均血球容積		**MTD**	(L. *Membrana tympani dextra*, right eardrum)　右耳膜
MD	Muscular dystrophy　肌肉失養症		**MTS**	(L. *Membrana tympani sinistra*, left eardrum)　左耳膜（膜鼓左）
Med.	Medical　內科		**mμ**	Millimicron (= nanometer)　奈米（十億分之一公尺）
mEq.	Milliequivalent　毫克當量			
meta	Metastasis　轉移			
MFT	Muscle function test　肌肉功能測試		# N	
Mg	Magnesium　鎂			
mg	Milligram　毫克		**N**	Nitrogen　氮
MG	Myasthenic gravis　重症肌無力		**NA**	Nurse anesthetist　麻醉護士
MH	Marital history　婚姻史		**NA**	Nursing assistant　助理護士，護佐
~	Menstrual history　月經史		**NaCl**	Sodium chloride　氯化鈉
MI	Mitral insufficiency　二尖瓣閉鎖不全		**NBN**	Newborn nursery　新生兒育嬰室
			NCC	Nursing clerical coordinator 護理督導
~	Myocardial infarction　心肌梗塞		**NCS**	Nerve conduction studies　神經傳導檢查
MIC	Minimum inhibitory concentration 最小抑制濃度		**NCV**	Nerve conductive velocity　神經傳導速率
MICU	Medical intensive care unit　內科加護病房		**NEC**	Necrotizing enterocolitis　壞死性腸炎
mix.	Mixture　混合			
ml	Milliliter　毫升		**ng**	Nanogram　十億分之一克；10^{-9}
MM	Medial meniscus　內側半月板		**NG**	Nasogastric　鼻餵食的
mm	Millimeter　公釐，毫米			

NICC	Neonatal intensive care center　新生兒加護中心	

NKA　Not known allergy　無已知過敏；過敏史不明

NLB　Needle liver biopsy　針刺肝臟活體組織切片

NMS　Neuroleptic malignant syndrome　抗精神病藥物惡性症候群

NMT　Nebulizing mist treatment　霧化噴霧治療

no.　(L. *Numerus*, the number of)　數目

NOA　Nurse obstetric assistant　產科護士助理

NP　New patient　新病人

~　Nuclear pharmacist　核醫藥師

~　Nurse practitioner　執業護士

NPC　Nasopharyngeal carcinoma　鼻咽癌

NPH　Normal pressure hydrocephalus　常壓性腦積水

NPO　(L. *Nulla per os*, nothing by mouth)　禁食

NS　Neurosurgery　神經外科

~　Normal saline(isotonic saline)　生理鹽水

NSAID　Nonsteroidal anti-inflammatory drug　非固醇類抗發炎藥物

NSD　Nasal septal deviation　鼻中隔彎曲

NSD　Normal spontaneous delivery　自然生產

NSICU　Neurosurgical intensive care unit　神經外科加護病房

NSP　Nurse specialist　臨床專科護理師

NSR　Normal sinus rhythm　正常竇性心律

NST　Non-stress test　無壓力試驗

NSU　Neurosurgical unit　神經外科病房

NSY　Nursery　育嬰室

NTC　Neurotrauma center　神經外傷中心

O

O₂　Oxygen　氧

OA　Osteoarthritis　骨關節炎

OAG　Open-angle glaucoma　開角型青光眼

OB　Occult blood　潛血

OB-Gyn or OBG　Obstetrics and gynecology　婦產科

OBS　Obstetrician, obstetrics　產科醫生，產科

~　Organic brain syndrome　器質性腦症候

OCD　Obsessive-compulsive disorder　強迫症

OCT　Oxytocin challenge test　催產素挑釁試驗

O.D.　(L. *Oculus dexter*, the eye of the right)　右眼

OGTT　Oral glucose tolerance test　口服葡萄糖耐受性試驗

OH　Occupational history　職業史

OHCA　Out of hospital cardiac arrest　到院前心跳停止

oint.　Ointment　軟膏

O.L.　(L. *Oculus laevus*, the eye of the left)　左眼

OM　Otitis media　中耳炎

OME　Otitis media effusion　積液性中耳炎

OMT　Osteopathic manipulative therapy　整骨手法治療

ON　Overnight　隔夜

OP　Operation　手術

O&P　Ova and Parasites　卵子和寄生蟲

OPD　Outpatient department　門診部

Oph.　Ophthalmology　眼科

OPU　Obstructive peptic ulcer　阻塞性消化性潰瘍

OREF　Open reduction with external fixation　開放性復位及外固定

ORIF　Open reduction with internal fixation　開放性復位及內固定

ORN　Operating room nurse　手術室護士

ORTHO	Orthopedics　骨科	
OS	(L. *Ocular sinistra*, left eye)　左眼	
~	Oral surgery　口腔外科	
~	Orthopedic surgery　整形外科	
OT	Occupational therapy　職能治療	
OTC	Over-the-counter　成藥	
OTR	Occupational therapist, registered 合格之職能治療師	
OU	(L. *Oculi unitas*, both eyes) 兩眼，雙眼	
~	Observation unit　觀察室	
OW	Once weekly　每週一次	
oz	Ounce　盎司（1/12 英磅）	

P

P	Parity　經產
~	Phosphorus　磷
~	Pressure　壓力
~	Pulse　脈搏
P&A	Percussion and auscultation 叩診與聽診
p.c.	(L. *Post cibum*, post meal)　飯後
p.o.	(L. *Per os*, by mouth)　口服
p.p.a.	(L. *Phiala prius agitate*)　瓶子先搖
p.r.	(L. *Pro recto*, via rectal)　經由直腸
p.r.n.	(L. *Pro re nata*, whenever necessary) 需要時
P/T	Phototherapy　光照療法
PA	Physician assistant　醫師助理
~	Posterior to anterior　由後至前
P$_A$CO$_2$	Alveolar carbon dioxide partial pressure　肺泡二氧化碳分壓
P$_a$CO$_2$	Arterial carbon dioxide partial pressure　動脈二氧化碳分壓
P$_a$O$_2$	Arterial oxygen partial pressure 動脈氧分壓
P$_A$O$_2$	Alveolar oxygen partial pressure 肺泡氧分壓
Pap. Smear	Papanicolaou smear　子宮頸抹片 檢查

PAR	Perennial allergic rhinitis　常年性過 敏性鼻炎
PAT	Paroxysmal cough　陣發性咳嗽
PCL	Posterior chamber lens　後防水晶體
PCN	Percutaneous nephrostomy　經皮腎 造口術
PCR	Polymerase chain reaction　聚合酶連 鎖反應
PCT	Penicillin test　盤尼西林測驗
PCV	Pneumococcal vaccine　肺炎球菌疫 苗
PD	Personality disorders　人格障礙
~	Pulmonary disease　肺疾病
PDA	Patent ductus arteriosus　開放性動 脈導管
PDL	Protein daily loss　全日蛋白質流失 量
PDR	Proliferative diabetic retinopathy 增生性糖尿病視網膜病變
PE	Physical examination　身體檢查
~	Pulmonary edema　肺水腫
~	Pulmonary embolist　肺栓塞
Ped.	Pediatrics　兒科
PES	Panendoscopy　胃鏡檢查
PET	Positron emission tomography 正子散射斷層攝影
PFT	Pulmonary function test　肺功能檢 查
pg	Picogram (= micromicrogram) 兆分之一公克（微微克）
PH	Personal history　個人史
P(M)H	Past(medical) history　過去病史
pH	Hydrogen ion concentration 氫離子濃度（酸鹼度）
PI	Pressent illness　現在病史
PID	Pelvic inflammatory disease 骨盆發炎症
pil.	Pill　丸劑
PK	Penetrating keratectomy　穿透性角 膜切削術
PKU	Phenylketonuria　苯酮尿症

PM.	(L. *Post meridiem*, afternoon) 午後	
PMN	Polymorphonuclear leukocyte 多型態核白血球	
PMS	Premenstrual syndrome　經前期症候群	
PN	Primary nurse　全責護理人員	
PND	Paroxysmal nocturnal dyspnea 陣發性夜間呼吸困難	
PNS	Peripheral nervous system　周圍神經系統	
POHR	Problem-oriented health recording 以健康問題為導向記錄法	
POMR	Problem-oriented medical recording 以醫療問題為導向記錄法	
POR	Post operative room　恢復室	
~	Problem-oriented recording 以問題為導向記錄法	
PP	Postpartum　產後的	
PP Cast	Plastic paris cast　整形硬石膏	
PPD	Purified protein derivative (tuberculin) 純化蛋白衍生物（結核菌素）	
PPH	Postpartum hemorrhage　產後出血	
ppm	Parts per million　百萬分之一部分	
PPU	Perforated peptic ulcer　穿孔性消化道潰瘍	
PR	Physical examination　身體檢查	
PROM	Premature rupture of the membranes 早期破水	
PS	Pulmonary valve stenosis　肺瓣膜狹窄	
PSA	Prostate specific antigen　前列腺特異性抗原	
PSG	Polysomnography　多導睡眠圖	
PSP	Progressive supranuclear palsy 進行性上眼神經核麻痺症	
PSVT	Paroxysmal supraventricular tachycardia　陣發性上心室心搏過速	
Psy.	Psychiatry　精神病學	
PT	Physical therapy　物理治療	
~	Prothrombin time　凝血酶原時間	

PTCA	Percutaneous transluminal cronary angioplasty　經皮穿腔冠狀動脈氣球擴張術
PTCD	Percutaneous transhepatic cholangia drainage　經皮穿肝膽道引流術
PTSD	Posttraumatic stress disorder 創傷後壓力症
PTT	Partial thromboplastin time 部分凝血激素時間
pulv.	(L. *Pulvis*, powder)　粉末
PV	Pervaginal　經由陰道
px.	Prognosis　預後

Q

Q	Every　每次
q2h	(L. *Quaque 2 hora*, every 2 hours) 每二小時
qh	(L. *Quaque hora*, every hour) 每小時
qs	(L. *Quantum sufficiat*, as much as is sufficient)　盡足量
qd	(L. *Quaque die*, everyday)　每天
qod	(L. *quaque other die*, every other day) 每隔一天
qoh	(L. *quaque other hora*, every other hour)　每隔一小時
qon	(L. *quaque other nocte*, every other night)　每隔一夜
qid	(L. *Quarter in Die*, four times a day) 一天四次

R

R	Resident　住院醫師
~	Respiration(rate)　呼吸（速率）
Ra	Radium　鐳
RA	Rheumatoid arthritis　風濕性關節炎
RAH	Radical abdominal hysterectomy 根治子宮切除術
RBC	Red blood cell　紅血球
RD	Retinal detachment　視網膜剝離

RDS	Respiratory distress syndrome 呼吸窘迫症候群	
RET	Rational-emotive therapy　理性情緒療法	
RF	Renal failure　腎衰竭	
RH⁺	Rhesus positive　Rh 陽性	
RHD	Rheumatoid heart disease　風濕性心臟病	
RICU	Respiratory intensive care unit 呼吸加護病房	
RIV	Radiculomyelopathy rupture into ventricle　神經根脊髓破裂進入腦室	
RK	Radical keratectomy　根除性角膜切除術	
RLQ	Right lower quadrant(abdomen) 右下象限	
RN	Rapid neuroleption　快速鎮靜療法	
~	Registered nurse　註冊護士	
RNA	Ribonucleic acid　核醣核酸	
R/O	Rule out　可能是，疑似，排除	
ROA	Right occiput anterior　右枕前位	
ROM	Range of motion　運動範圍	
ROP	Right occiput posterior　右枕後位	
ROT	Right occiput transverse　右枕橫位	
RPG	Retrograde pyelogram　逆行性腎盂造影照片	
Rph	Registered pharmacist　註冊藥劑師	
RR	Recovery room　恢復室	
RRT	Registered respiratory therapist 註冊呼吸治療師	
RT	Radiotherapy　放射線療法	
RT	Rapid tranquilization　快速鎮靜療法	
~	Respiratory therapist　呼吸治療師	
RUQ	Right upper quadrant(abdomen) 右上象限	
℞	Prescription　處方	

S

S	Without　沒有	
~	Surgery　外科	
SA	Spontaneous abortion　自發性流產	
SAH	Subarachnoid hemorrhage　蜘蛛膜下腔出血	
Sao₂	Arterial oxygen saturation　動脈氧飽和度	
SARS	Severe acute respiratory syndrome 嚴重急性呼吸道症候群	
SAS	Sleep apnea syndrome　睡眠呼吸暫停症候群	
SBE	Subacute bacterial endocarditis 亞急性細菌性心內膜炎	
SBS	Shaken baby syrdrome　搖晃嬰兒症候群	
SC	Subcutaneous(injection)　皮下的（注射）	
SCC	Squamous cell carcinoma　鱗狀細胞癌	
SCI	Spina cord injury　脊髓損傷	
SDH	Subdural hematoma　硬膜下血腫	
semih.	(L. *Semihora*, every half hour)　每半小時	
SGA	Small for gestational age　胎兒大小不足妊娠期	
SI	International system of units 國際單位	
SIDS	Sudden infant death syndrome 嬰兒猝死症候群	
SJS	Stevens-Johnson syndrome　史蒂芬症候群	
SL	Sublingual　舌下的	
SLE	Systemic lupus erythematosus 全身性紅斑性狼瘡	
SMA	Spinal muscle atrophy　脊髓肌肉萎縮	
SN	Student nurse　護生	
SOB	Short(shortness)of breath 短（急促）呼吸	
sol.	Solution　溶液	

SOM	Serous otitis media　漿液性中耳炎		**Td**	Tetanus toxoid(vaccine)　破傷風菌疫苗
SOR	Source-oriented recording　以資料來源為導向記錄法		**TF**	Tetralogy of Fallot　法洛氏四重畸形
s.o.s.	(L. *Si opus sit*, if need)　如有所需		**TG**	Triglyceride　三酸甘油酯
S/P	Post-surgical　手術後		**TGV**	Transposition of great vessels 大血管轉位
sp.gr.	Specific gravity　比重		**THR**	Total hip replacement　全髖關節骨換術
SPECT	Single photon emission computery 單一光子放射斷層檢查		**TI**	Tricuspid insufficiency　三尖瓣閉鎖不全
ss.	Semi or semisse　一半		**TIA**	Transient ischemic attack　暫時性腦缺血發作
SSRI	Selective serotonin reuptake inhibitor 選擇性血清素在攝取抑制劑		**TICU**	Thoracic intensive care unit 胸腔心臟血管加護中心
SSS	Sick sinus syndrome　病態竇房結症候群		**tid**	(L. *ter in die*, 3 times a day)　一天三次
st	(L. *Statim*, immediately)　立刻		**tine**	Tincture　酊劑
staph	*Staphylococcus*　葡萄球菌		**TKR**	Total knee replacement 全膝關節骨換術
STH	Subtotal hysterectomy　次全子宮切除術		**TL**	Tubal ligation　輸卵管結紮
strep	*Streptococcus*　鏈球菌		**TNF**	Tumor necrosis factor　腫瘤凋亡因子
STS	Serologic test for syphilis　梅毒血清學試驗		**TOA**	Tubo-ovarian abscess　輸卵管卵巢膿腫
SUI	Stress urinary incontinence　壓力性尿失禁		**TP**	Total protein　蛋白質總量
supp.	Suppositoria　坐藥，塞劑		**TP**	Total parenteral nutrition　全靜脈營養法
Susp	Suspension　懸浮液		**TR**	Tricuspid regurgitation　三尖瓣返流
s.y.r.	Syrup　糖漿		**TS**	Tricuspid stenosis　三尖瓣狹窄
			TT	Tuberculin test　結核菌素測驗
			TTH	Transfusion transmitted hepatitis 輸血後肝炎

T

T	Tablespoon　一湯匙		**TURBT**	Transurethral resection of bladder tumor　經尿道膀胱腫瘤切除術
~	Temperature　溫度		**TURP**	Transurethral resection of the prostate 經尿道前列腺切除術
tab	Tablet(s)　碇劑		**TX**	Treatment　治療
TAE	Transarterial embolization　經動脈栓塞			
TAH	Total abdominal hysterectomy 經腹部子宮全切除術			
TB	Tuberculosis　結核病			
TC	Turn cough　反覆咳嗽			
TCC	Transitional cell carcinoma　轉移性細胞癌			
TD	Tardive dyskinesia　遲發性運動障礙			

U

UA	Urine analysis	尿液分析
UC	Ulcerative colitis	潰瘍性結腸炎
~	Ureter catheterization	輸尿管導管
UGI	Upper gastrointestinal	上腸胃道
UPJ	Ureteropelvic junction	輸尿管腎盂連接處
URI	Upper respiratory infection	上呼吸道感染
Uro.	Urology	泌尿科
US	Ultrasound	超音波
USD	Ventricular septal defect	心室中隔缺損
USI	Urinary stress incontinence	壓力性尿失禁
USO	Unilateral salpingo-oophorectomy	單側輸卵管卵巢切除術
UTI	Urinary tract infection	泌尿道感染
UV	Ultraviolet	紫外線的
UVJ	Ureterovesical junction	輸尿管膀胱連接部
μ	Micro-, micron	「微一」，百萬分之一
μg	Microgram	微克（百萬分之一公克）

V

VD	Venereal disease	性病
VDRL	Venereal disease research laboratories	梅毒血清檢驗

VED	Vacuum extration delivery	真空吸出分娩
Vf	Ventricular fibrillation	心室纖維性顫動
VF	Ventricular flutter	心室撲動
VHD	Valvular heart disease	瓣膜性心臟病
V-P shunt	Ventricular peritoneal shunt	腦室腹膜腔分流
VPC	Ventricular permature contraction	心室早期收縮
VS	Visiting staff	主治醫師
~	Vital signs	生命徵象
VSD	Ventricular septal defect	心室中隔缺損
VT	Ventricular tachyarrhythmia	心室性頻脈

W

WBC & DC	White blood count and differential count	白血球計數與血球計數
WHO	World health organization	世界衛生組織
WNL	Within normal limits	在正常範圍內
wt	Weight	重量

X

XR　X-ray　Ｘ光

Y

y/o　Year(s) old, year(s)　年齡

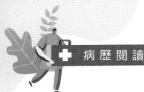

 參考資料 REFERENCES

王美綺(2021)・紀錄，於王桂芸總校閱，*基本護理學*（九版）・永大。

王琦、廖梅珍(2001)・經腹腔鏡卵巢切除術臨床路徑實施之成效・*長庚護理*，*12*(1)，23-29。

王璟璇、陳慧敏、簡芷茵、侯宜菁、楊金蘭(2019)・*病歷閱讀*（二版）・華杏。

江鴻華、江銘酌(2002)・胃食道逆流的中西醫治療・*台灣中醫臨床醫學會*，*8*(4)，40-46。

李佩育、溫孟娟、劉怡秀、劉明德、吳寶觀、沈燕芬、張淑女、蔡秀美、劉佩青、曾翊瑄、孫淑敏(2021)・*醫護專用術語*（五版）・華格那。

李皎正(2021)・*常用醫護術語*（六版）・華杏。

杜金芝(2010)・*台灣胃食道逆流的發生率及危險因子之探討*・國立高雄海洋科技大學。

汪昂(1694)・*本草備要*・啟業書局。

卓妙如、陳佳鳳、趙宏明(2001)・臨床路徑照護流程及成效探討以小兒腹股溝修補術為例・*領導護理*，*4*(2)，37-44。

周守民、顏妙芬(2002)・資訊時代中的臨床路徑發展・*台灣醫學*，*6*(2)，251-255。

林宛儀、周恬弘、黃勝雄(2002)・從病患滿意度的角度探討臨床路徑實施成效－以某區域醫院為例・*醫院*，*35*(5)，34-43。

徐秀栞(2020)・紀錄，*新編基本護理學——學理與技術*（三版）・新文京。

徐南麗、賴正芬、謝美玲、廖惠娥、林碧珠(2002)・比較實施臨床路徑前後之護理品質・*慈濟護理雜誌*，*1*(2)，77-86。

啟業書局(1988)・*中醫病因病機學*・啟業書局。

張吉仰(2008)・胃食道逆流症與巴瑞特氏食道・*義大醫訊*，*4*(6)，8-12。

張伯臾(2010)・*中醫內科學*・知音出版社。

陳建如、曾惠明、鄭錦翔(2001)・臨床路徑使用於卵巢或輸卵管切除術：連續實施十二個月的描述性分析・*醫院*，*34*，14-21。

廖思嘉、葉宏仁、柯忠旺、連漢仲、張繼森(2010)・胃食道逆流疾病之處置現況・*內科學誌*，*21*(6)，381-390。

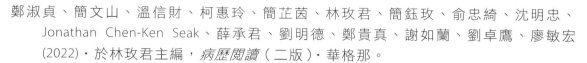

鄭淑貞、簡文山、溫信財、柯惠玲、簡芷茵、林玫君、簡鈺玫、俞忠綺、沈明忠、Jonathan Chen-Ken Seak、薛承君、劉明德、鄭貴真、謝如蘭、劉卓鷹、廖敏宏 (2022)・於林玫君主編，*病歷閱讀*（二版）・華格那。

蕭嘉琪、朱苓珍、廖姿婷、邱燕甘、李素宏、武佳縈(2006)・提升護理人員執行剖腹產臨床路徑之完整率・*長庚護理*，17(4)，445-465。

Joyce, Y. J., & Jim, K. (2010). *Pediatric Nursing.* Demystified McGraw-Hill Companies, Inc.

Peter, J., & Kahrilas, M. D. (n. d.). *Clinical manifestations and diagnosis of gastroesophageal reflux in adults.* http://www.uptodate.com/contents/acid-reflux-gastroesophageal-reflux-disease-in-adults-beyond-the-basics

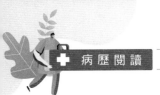
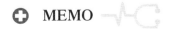

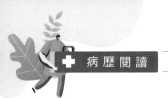

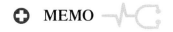 MEMO

MEMO

國家圖書館出版品預行編目資料

病歷閱讀 / 劉明德，蔡玟蕙，郭彥志，黃盈禎，林玫君，
鄭雅敏，徐玉珍，張玠，陳寶如，陳勝美，薛承君，Jonathan
Chen-Ken Seak，王守玉，卓淑美，李正喆，魏鈴穎，曹
永昌，謝瓊慧，梁繼權，謝如蘭，張皓翔，潘昭貴，林
鳳映，陳麗琴，陳麗貞，陳滄山，陳瑋芬，周志和，釋
高上，王惠芳，李惠萍，李昭螢等編著. – 第六版. – 新
北市：新文京開發出版股份有限公司, 2023.06
面；　公分

ISBN　978-986-430-929-0（平裝）

1. CST: 病歷　2. CST: 病歷管理

415.206　　　　　　　　　　　　　　　　112007952

病歷閱讀（第六版）　　　　　　　（書號：B338e6）

審 訂 者	徐會棋	胡月娟	李中一	鍾國彪	張銘峰	林清華
編 著 者	劉明德	蔡玟蕙	郭彥志	黃盈禎	林玫君	鄭雅敏
	徐玉珍	張　玠	陳寶如	陳勝美	薛承君	
	Jonathan Chen-Ken Seak			王守玉	卓淑美	李正喆
	魏鈴穎	曹永昌	謝瓊慧	梁繼權	謝如蘭	張皓翔
	潘昭貴	林鳳映	陳麗琴	陳麗貞	陳滄山	陳瑋芬
	周志和	釋高上	王惠芳	李惠萍	李昭螢	

出 版 者　新文京開發出版股份有限公司
地　　　址　新北市中和區中山路二段 362 號 9 樓
電　　　話　(02) 2244-8188（代表號）
Ｆ　Ａ　Ｘ　(02) 2244-8189
郵　　　撥　1958730-2
第 四 版　西元 2017 年 8 月 15 日
第 五 版　西元 2019 年 11 月 30 日
第 六 版　西元 2023 年 6 月 2 日

New Wun Ching Developmental Publishing Co., Ltd.
New Age · New Choice · The Best Selected Educational Publications—NEW WCDP

新文京開發出版股份有限公司

NEW WCDP

新世紀‧新視野‧新文京 ― 精選教科書‧考試用書‧專業參考書